Demonstrating Care

The Art of Integrative Nursing

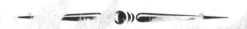

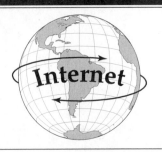

Demonstrating Care

The Art of Integrative Nursing

Martha Libster, MS, RN

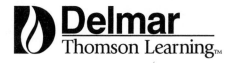

Africa • Australia • Canada • Denmark • Japan • Mexico • New Zealand • Philippines
Puerto Rico • Singapore • Spain • United Kingdom • United States

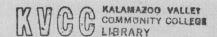

NOTICE TO THE READER

Publisher does not warrant or guarantee any of the products described herein or perform any independent analysis in connection with any of the product information contained herein. Publisher does not assume, and expressly disclaims, any obligation to obtain and include information other than that provided to it by the manufacturer.

The reader is expressly warned to consider and adopt all safety precautions that might be indicated by the activities herein and to avoid all potential hazards. By following the instructions contained herein, the reader willingly assumes all risks in connection with such instructions.

The publisher makes no representation or warranties of any kind, including but not limited to, the warranties of fitness for particular purpose or merchantability, nor are any such representations implied with respect to the material set forth herein, and the publisher takes no responsibility with respect to such material. The publisher shall not be liable for any special, consequential, or exemplary damages resulting, in whole or part, from the readers' use of, or reliance upon, this material.

Delmar Staff:
Business Unit Director: William Brottmiller
Product Development Manager: Marion Waldman
Product Development Editor: Jill Rembetski
Editorial Assistant: Penny Cartwright
Executive Marketing Manager: Dawn Gerrain
Art and Design Coordinator: Rich Killar
Cover Design: Joanne Beckman Design

ISBN: 0-7668-1766-0

Dedication

This book is dedicated to Florence Nightingale, the fiery, mystical mother of a holistic, caring profession. It is dedicated to all the caring souls who have and will continue to follow the light of Florence's lamp in the new millennium, with all of its challenges, opportunities, joys, and mystery.

On a personal note, this book is dedicated to my beloved Harold whose daily care for my body and soul has kept me going, and in whom I have found an extraordinary, tender-hearted being so receptive to my own demonstrations of love and care.

Contents

PART THREE: Caring Modalities: Nursing and Complementary Therapies   93

PART FOUR: The Evolution of Nursing Practice   205

Foreword

This new work by Martha Libster offers a hopeful framework for an authentic yet integrated practice model that restores caring in the midst of contemporary demands. *Demonstrating Care: The Art of Integrative Nursing* is a comprehensive book that makes new connections between nursing within the biomedical world and its integrative developments that allow theory and action to comingle for new reasons, resulting in specific and explicit models of caring in practice. Such directions integrate past and present, science and art, and old and new paradigm thinking, leading to redefinitions and new openings for an expanded practice of caring, now intersecting with mind-body medicine and the latest developments in complementary and alternative practices.

Libster's approach is highly integrative, bringing together historical understanding with the most contemporary and futuristic thinking in nursing and the broader health field. The perspective of this text is grounded in the discipline of nursing, yet also is grounded in professional practice for a new era. Areas such as art and science, communication, relationship, reframed nursing fundamentals, touch therapies, healing dynamics, and the body as energy are located within the most progressive thinking, beliefs, and scientific paradigms in the field, as well as timeless themes in nursing's past.

The result is *Demonstrating Care: The Art of Integrative Nursing*, a relevant book for educators and clinicians, for generalist and advanced practitioners. It serves as a map of nursing's evolving practices and hopes, while offering a blueprint for the future: a future that is integrative, transformed, and encompassing of caring and healing knowledge and practices, waiting to be fully actualized. This work serves as a comprehensive educational and professional framework whereby Nightingale's paradigm for nursing is more capable of being actualized. This work informs contemporary nursing, whereby nurses are helped to integrate nursing's past, present, and future into a coherent advanced professional *nursing* model, reflecting the highest level of caring and healing practices.

Jean Watson, PhD, RN, FAAN, HNC
University of Colorado Health Sciences Center
School of Nursing/International Center for
Integrative Caring Practices
Denver, Colorado

Preface

This text is written for nurses who *wonder* about complementary therapies and how they relate to nursing practice. I have *wondered* for a long time about complementary therapies myself. When I began my professional career in dance and movement therapy, "complementary therapies" didn't exist, at least in name. I was not called a complementary therapy practitioner. Yet, today, the public cannot seem to get enough of these sometimes ancient, sometimes contemporary, healing modalities. Are nurses able to meet the public's demand for these caring modalities and if so, how? This book shows that throughout history, nurses have been providers of many of the caring modalities now known as complementary therapies.

Historically, caring modalities in nursing, in particular, and health care, in general, are developed as the *art* of the professional practice. Yet the largest growth in health care around the world, even in developing nations, has occurred more in the area of biomedical and technical science. During the past decade in nursing, there has been a tremendous emphasis on the mastery of biomedical and technical skills and less emphasis on the development of the caring arts or *fundamentals* of nursing such as creating a healing environment with the patient, providing healing through touch, providing nourishment, engaging in communication, and using energy for healing. The public has noticed that nurses have steered away from offering fundamental caring modalities that have been associated for years with "good nursing care." The public has turned to the practitioner of complementary therapies for many of the caring modalities that nurses provided as a matter of routine.

Fundamental caring modalities such as feeding a patient or giving a massage are what nurses do to create healing relationships with patients. Nurses are caring people. What makes each nurse unique is the way she demonstrates care to a patient. Because my education is in dance and movement therapy, I am fascinated by the way people communicate their feelings through actions. Since becoming a nurse many years ago, I have realized that through the actions, tasks, or modalities we use in nursing, we not only convey our caring, compassionate feelings, but also we are able to create healing relationships with patients. Many present-day nursing tasks have evolved technologically but not necessarily artistically. Many of the simple tasks such as bathing, feeding, and talking with patients are now seen as mundane and something that a nurse should delegate.

Having come to the nursing profession from another healing art, dance, I have wondered what would become of the art of nursing as the profession became more and more focused on the world of technology. I wondered if nurses would have the desire to find a balance between providing care that included both technical, biomedical skills and caring modalities. I wrote this book in response to the trend I perceived in health care, in general, and in nursing, in particular. It is not too late for nurses to take notice of this trend and explore the possibilities for greater integration of their biomedical skills with fundamental caring modalities.

Organization

There are four parts in this book. Part One helps the reader explore the influences of the biomedical world as well as the possibilities for integrating biomedical and caring skills in nursing practice. The concept of integrative nursing is defined. Part Two takes the philosophical and theoretical concept of caring into the realm of action—*demonstrating* care, past, present, and future. The reader is offered an opportunity in Chapter 5 for reflection on five aspects of demonstrating care. Part Three begins by addressing the connection between nursing fundamentals and complementary therapies. Chapters 7–11 give the reader an opportunity to explore each of the five categories of nursing fundamentals or modalities and their present-day connection with complementary therapies. The science and art of each modality is addressed. In Part Four, Chapters 12–14, readers then take their understanding of integrative nursing, how they and others demonstrate care, and complementary therapies, and are encouraged to begin to imagine the evolution of nursing practice. A visual guideline, the Healing Relationship Model, is presented as a guideline for integrative nursing practice.

Features

Throughout *Demonstrating Care,* there are photographs depicting the way nurses have demonstrated care throughout history, including nurses providing complementary therapies. All of the photos express relationship with patients.

One of the primary themes of this book is the development of the healing relationship as the foundation for integrative nursing practice. The style of this book reflects this theme. I use nurses' narratives from their experience of demonstrating care as well as personal experience to help the reader connect with and form a relationship with the concepts in the book. Pictures, stories, and models are used to assist the reader in identifying ways to use this material in practice. Just as nurses in the new millennium can ground their practice in the development of the healing relationship, so too must the nursing textbooks of the new millennium engage the reader in a relationship for a fuller, perhaps more meaningful, learning experience to occur. It is my hope that you will find this to be so with this book.

Audience

This book was written for all nurses who are trying to integrate complementary therapies into their biomedical practice. It is also written for the novice nurse, for experienced nurses who are reevaluating their practice, and for those who may not be nurses but who feel they could benefit from understanding more about nursing and/or demonstrating care. This book can be used in nursing fundamentals and theory courses especially when caring theory is studied. Other courses for which this book can be used at all levels are complementary therapies courses and "health and healing" courses. This book can also be used by organizations to promote creativity and a deeper integration of caring and biomedical skills and modalities by their health care providers.

Acknowledgments

I wish to thank the following people with all my heart who have so generously demonstrated their care for this project: Betty Neuman; Jean Watson; Marlaine Smith; Sally Phillips; Marilyn Doenges; Mindy Green; Usha Varma; Dana Murphy-Parker; Carolyn Cummings; Michele Bowman; Debbie Doberson; Carma Lovely; Kathleen Brockman; Barbara Fine; Dorothy Schwabb; Kathleen Christiansen; Kathi Lersh and the Children's Hospital of Denver; Pat Nelson; Lauren Clark; Sandra Jeanne Fucci; Betsy Weiss and the Center for the Study of the History of Nursing; Jane Hoffmann; Janice Haugen, "the ten nurse experts"; S.K.; L.M.V.; M.M.; E.M.; N.R., and C.L.K.. And a special thanks to my mom, Connie Chapman, and to Marion Waldman, Jill Rembetski, and Penny Cartwright for their vision and support.

I would also like to thank the following reviewers:

Karen Aiken, RN, MSN, CNOR
Department of Nursing
University of Hartford
West Hartford, CT

JoAnn L. Ercums
Assistant Professor
College of Nursing
University of South Alabama
Fairhope, AL

Carol Harrison, BSN, MA, MSN, EdD
Chair, Division of Nursing
Spring Hill College
Mobile, AL

Kathryn A. Lauchner, PhD, RN
Professor of Nursing
Austin Community College
Austin, TX

Lynn Rew, EdD, RNC, HNC, FAAN
Associate Professor
School of Nursing
The University of Texas at Austin
Austin, TX

Marlaine Smith, PhD, RN
Department of Nursing
University of Colorado
Denver, CO

PART ONE

INTEGRATIVE NURSING

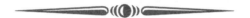

"THERE'S NOTHING NEW UNDER THE SUN." THAT'S WHAT A
wonderful teacher of mine told me years ago in a class
in which I was to "learn" how to choreograph dances. I'd been
choreographing and performing my own dances since I was seven
years old. Then I went to school to organize and develop my craft.
That's when I realized that "art" is not about "creating something."
It's about creating something *anew,* in a new way, my way. So as I write
this book I know that what I have to say probably is not really new
or even unique to myself. For history often repeats itself with just a
subtle change here and there.

This is how I feel about the healing arts in general and what are being called "complementary and alternative" therapies in particular. There really isn't anything "new under the sun" when we look at the list of complementary therapies. Many of these therapies have been around for centuries. And most importantly to the nursing profession, many of the therapies and modalities listed as complementary and alternative medicine—massage, nutrition, and hydrotherapy, to name just a few—have been part of nursing care for centuries.

Complementary therapies have been part of medicine, too. It is not the purpose of this book to claim that any of the complementary therapies are the domain of nursing alone. Many of the complementary therapies address lifestyle practices that are addressed in most, if not all, areas of the healing arts.

The purpose of this book is threefold. The first is to discuss the importance of nurses demonstrating caring and gaining a deeper understanding of the therapeutic use of self in their healing relationship with patients. The second is to define integrative nursing as the creation of evolving, healing relationships with patients in which the nurse observes the patients' needs for greater harmony and balance in their lives and then addresses those needs by offering care that is a holistic blend of biomedical and caring skills. And the third is to offer a greater understanding of five areas of complementary therapies—touch, creating a healing environment, nutrition, communication, and the use of energy for therapy—and how nurses have historically used these modalities in practice as well as how we can begin to develop them as part of nursing practice in the new millennium.

Demonstrating Care

The way nurses demonstrate care is influenced by many social, environmental, and cultural factors. The way nurses as individual practitioners demonstrate care is influenced by who they are as people. How people demonstrate care to each other is one way they manifest their personality and the essence of their being. How nurses demonstrate care is as unique as the human beings they are. Caring is communicated through our actions. Think about those who have cared for you. Have you ever been in a relationship with a family member or friend in which the person tells you often how much she cares for you, even loves you, but you just don't believe it deep inside? You find that her behavior toward you just doesn't seem to match the words she says. Your head tells you that she "must love you." You may even know that she wants to love you, but you don't feel the love or see it demonstrated so explicitly that there is no question in your mind or heart that she truly cares for you.

Demonstrating love or caring feelings for another human being is not always as easy as we might think. Different people demonstrate caring in different ways based on their own life experiences in intimate relationships. Demonstrating caring involves a very deep level of intimacy and effort on the caregiver's part. Imagine for a moment a scenario in which a nurse attempts to comfort a patient who is sad and lonely. The nurse sits beside the patient, doesn't look at him and says, "You know, I really care about you." What do you imagine the patient's response will be?

Another nurse might approach the same situation in a different way. This nurse approaches the patient with eye contact, if culturally appropriate, and puts her hand on the patient's shoulder and says, "You know, I really care about you. Can you tell me what's going on?" A third nurse might be less direct. She might spend time finding out what the patient really likes, perhaps a special food. The nurse then makes sure that the patient receives the special food at a time when the patient is hungry. She watches the response.

Which way of letting the patient know that he is cared for would have "worked" for you? How do you effectively communicate your true caring feelings? Does the method in which caring is demonstrated affect the patient's perception of being cared for? Through observation and experience, I can say that it truly does.

Demonstrating care to another human being involves communication—effective communication. Some people really appreciate a comforting word. Some people need more. Some need to *feel* and *see* the demonstration of the caring feelings. They perceive caring through gesture, posture, and body language more than through a kind word.

For decades, professional nursing has been associated with the act of caring. Nurses are very different in how they demonstrate their caring feelings to patients. Some nurses are comfortable with very intimate, caring relationships with patients and some are not. Some nurses put a lot of effort into the care of their patients and some do not. This variation in practice is influenced by factors such as culture, family experience, personal healing experience, and physical and emotional well-being, to name a few.

Nurses can develop a range or levels of caring behaviors regardless of what their particular preference and level of comfort is when entering the profession. For example, the nurse who is concerned about a patient who has been told by her physician that she is dying may not be able to verbalize her concerns to the patient because she is overwhelmed by her own fear of death. The nurse can be taught how to deal with her fear as well as how to interact with a patient at this stage of illness. Being able to interact with patients in this way takes tremendous skill and flexibility; it also takes creativity.

How nurses creatively demonstrate caring is the art of nursing. It's the beauty of nursing. It's also the science of nursing. This book is about the creative nursing activity of demonstrating care. It is written on the premise that the men and women who enter the nursing profession are genuinely caring, empathetic individuals who love people. This book is also written on the premise that there is a foundational understanding to the art and science of *demonstrating* care to others that must be taught to nurses. There is no "cookbook" approach to how nurses *should* demonstrate caring.

That's not what this book is about. This book is meant to be a guide, an opportunity, for nurses to begin to explore, in an in-depth way, the creative part of "how" and "what" they do every day in their caring work.

This book discusses the various caring modalities available to nurses that have been used for decades in the act of caring. It is my hope that in discussing the ways in which nurses demonstrate caring, and the modalities that can be used in doing so, nurses will feel free to develop their own unique style of caring practice that is energizing.

Professional nurses demonstrate who they are as healers in their *relationships* with patients. Part of the art of nursing is learning how to create healing relationships that demonstrate care. I once worked with an older nurse in a rural health clinic. On one of her cabinets she had a small poster that said, "Nobody knows what I do until I don't do it." This is true about the subtlest of caring professions. It speaks of nursing. My hope is that you find this book informative and inspiring and that it allows you the space of a precious moment of self-reflection on the importance of the healing relationships you create, as well as the importance of the seemingly insignificant things you do every day, all day long.

Integrative Nursing

Integrative nursing is defined throughout this book as an ongoing creative process. In a high-tech world, it is no longer sufficient to just say that we are a caring profession. We need to *be* a caring profession. The philosophy and practice of integrative nursing are discussed in detail in hope that you might realize by example that you don't have to choose *between* the biomedical world and caring modalities. Our patients need both. My hope is that you will be inspired to find your own way, as I continue to find mine, to integrating all that you have learned of the biomedical world, with all of its science and wonder, with all that you are as a caring, compassionate nurse and human being.

Complementary Therapies

The information in this book on complementary therapies draws from my years of working with a multidisciplinary group of health practitioners in a practice that integrated many complementary therapies with conventional biomedical practices. My goal is not to provide answers for how you can integrate caring modalities such as complementary therapies into your practice. That would be stealing your thunder! Instead, in addition to providing examples from my practice, I describe many caring and complementary therapies, why and how they have been used historically, and how they are currently used in *nursing* practice so that you can choose, if you haven't already, the modalities that work best for you in developing healing relationships with patients.

This book presents the stories or narratives of ten nurses from ten different specialty areas of nursing. Five of the nurses are retired after many years of nursing service and five are currently in practice. They were asked how they have demonstrated caring over the years. A number of important themes emerged from their responses. These themes can help to further illuminate nurses' caring service to humanity. Our profession is rich with caring experiences and expertise. As you read my stories, and those of ten other colleagues, my hope is that you will remember your own stories of the ways you have demonstrated care as a nurse and healer.

My story begins with dance. Having been a dancer my whole life, I grew up in a world of nonverbal expression. How people demonstrate caring to other people has always been of greater importance to me than the words of caring, which can be empty when not attached to a genuine and heartfelt act of caring.

As a professional nurse, caring has taken on greater significance for me than I ever imagined in my younger days when I learned the golden rule of "Do unto others as you would have them do unto you." This is such a simple, basic admonition that it is stated in many ways, in many cultures. Yet, I've learned throughout my nursing career that many people do not seem to know how they would have others treat them and care for them. Many people do not know how to really care for themselves. There is a huge range of abuses and neglects of the body, mind, and spirit in many cultures. I've sometimes wondered where humanity would be if we truly followed the golden rule. The key word is to treat others as you *would* have them treat you. Perhaps the meaning of the golden rule is to treat others in a way that is imagined as the best way to be treated, maybe even the most caring way to be treated.

A nurse's challenge is to demonstrate caring of the body, mind, and spirit that is exemplary and maybe even ideal. A nurse's calling is to treat fellow humans with the dignity and respect she may never have experienced from others in a world where the golden rule may or may not exist even though we'd like to think that it does. This book is about the challenge and calling a nurse accepts on a daily basis. It is about the way a nurse demonstrates caring and, historically, how these quiet demonstrations of compassion and love have led a profession to world recognition as a caring profession.

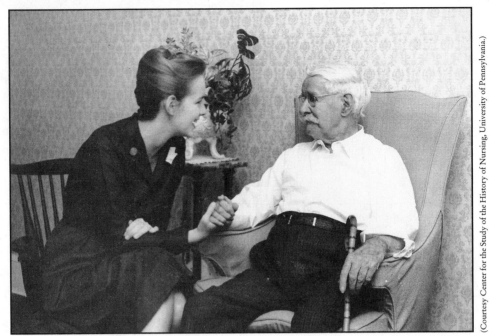

Nurse visitor, 1964

I knew nothing of books when I came forth from the womb

of my mother, and I shall die without books;

I shall die with another human hand in my own.

—MARTIN BUBER

CHAPTER 1

Nursing in a Biomedical World

I love nursing. I love walking beside people who are trying to understand how their bodies work or why their bodies aren't working. I love to listen to people talk about their lives and what health and illness mean to them. I love caring for infants and marveling at the greatest work of art and science on the planet—human life itself. I guess it all boils down to loving life with all its ups and downs and "in-betweens." Being a nurse gives me the opportunity to be at the heart of the living experience, where I can witness the lived experience of others.

I love the human body. Always have. When I was a young girl, I loved my Invisible Woman model. I painted her organs and put the model together. I have often sat in complete wonder at the workings of the body and how delicate the balance of life really is. I also grew up in a home where the human spirit was a major focus of our daily life. My father and my mother raised us in a home of ritual and community service.

I also experienced the human spirit in the art of dance. I was classically trained in the Denishawn dance method beginning at age seven. Dance, as an art form, is an expression or demonstration of the human spirit and emotions, using the body as the instrument. Movement has always been my preferred method of communication as well as the way I experience my world. Therefore, my understanding of the human body, spirit, and emotions has always come through movement, action, or behavior.

Nursing practice has allowed me to explore my understanding of the connectedness of body, mind, and spirit in myself as a caregiver as well as in the people I have cared for. It is in the act of caring, the demonstration of caring—the "dance" of caring, if you will—that I have found the heart of what I call integrative nursing.

Integrative nursing combines the medical profession's biomedical understanding of disease and treatment with the caring behaviors and treatments that have been part of nursing practice throughout history. A scientific and artistic synergy is reached when biomedical and caring skills are combined. The concept of synergy is that the whole is greater than the sum of the parts. In integrative nursing, a plan of care is developed in which the goal is the creation of a unique healing relationship between a nurse and a patient. Although this book will refer to the patient, it should be understood that the patient can indeed be, and often is, more than one person. The plan of care chosen by the nurse and patient draws upon both the biomedical and caring skills of the nurse. Integrative nursing is a process of helping a patient find greater health, harmony, and balance through the use of both highly technical biomedical skills and sometimes very basic human caring skills. As nurses begin the process of integration, they often find that their biomedical skills have received greater emphasis. This is not surprising because nursing has been closely associated with the biomedical model of health care, especially since the end of World War II.

Many nurses are now evaluating how the biomedical paradigm fits with nursing practice in the twenty-first century. Sister Rosemary Donley writes that nursing is at a "crossroads, a decision point for patients, providers, financiers, managers, system architects and policymakers" (1996, p. 325). She says that the "dialog at the crossroads challenges the very principles which have undergird America's health care delivery system and calls for a rethinking of America's social policies and the role of government in enacting and implementing them" (Donley, 1996, p. 325). The changes and challenges in the health care system could be described as an identity crisis, a time for redefining self. Western health care has come to be known throughout the world for its leadership in biotechnology and the use of drugs and surgery to treat illness.

What has been developed medically in Western countries is nothing short of miraculous, and yet no health care system is perfect for all situations and all people at all times. Questions at the "crossroads" are starting to arise about the delivery of health care, the health professions and their roles, patient needs, and on and on. Nurses at the crossroads are evaluating the culture of nursing, what is unique about nursing practice, and what the profession will be doing in the new millennium.

Although professional nurses have been developing their scientific and biomedical skills since the mid-1900s, the basics of nursing care have been passed to paraprofessionals. Many patients search for comfort measures outside of nursing. They have turned to practitioners of complementary therapies. Many of the modalities and treatments provided by alternative and complementary therapists were once performed by nurses as part of basic nursing practice. For example, nurses used to give back rubs as part of evening care. Nurses have questioned the efficacy and importance of the back rub and have stopped the practice in many facilities. Many organizations are now hiring massage therapists to treat their patients. There seems to be a decision by some nursing leaders that nurses are needed to do "more important duties" than massage. Some patients say that they do not expect back rubs from nurses anymore. Nurses are faced with the decision whether to continue to turn the focus of nursing education and practice away from caring modalities, such as massage, or to determine through research how the use of these historic comfort measures can best be utilized in an integrated nursing practice for healing and health promotion. Nurses are evaluating whether these caring modalities might be needed now more than ever in today's high-tech and high-stress world where the emphasis of health care has been the development and promotion of biomedicine.

Years ago I had a professional experience that forever changed my understanding of the importance of nursing in a biomedical world. I was caring for a woman who had given birth to a healthy infant by cesarean section the day before. She was fine the morning I assumed care for her, but that afternoon things changed quickly. She had been sitting up in her chair and doing well. After lunch, her family came to find me to tell me that she was shaking uncontrollably. I went to her room, where I found her conscious and feverish. I took her vital signs and found that her temperature was 105 degrees and both her systolic and diastolic blood pressures were very high. I called for the physician on the unit. What occurred from this point on is ingrained in my memory.

While monitoring the patient's vital signs, I put cool towels around her ankles to keep the fever out of her head, and I tried to give her IV fluids. The IV fluids would not run in. I gave the woman medication for the fever as per doctor's orders, then I took her hand and had her take slow, deep breaths so she would stop hyperventilating. The physician stood and watched what we were doing. He could do nothing at that time for the patient except order lab tests. I could see he was desperately trying to understand what was going wrong with this patient. After leaving for a moment to get something for the patient, I came back to the room to find the physician holding the patient's hand and encouraging her to breathe slowly as I had been doing. As quickly as they had come on, the symptoms went away. The patient's fever and blood pressure returned to normal. The labs were drawn, and the IV started to run in. There were no other occurrences that day.

The episode taught me a valuable lesson. At times, biomedical science has much to offer patients, including saving their lives. But at other times biomedicine fails patients miserably. Even the most basic nursing interventions are useful to patients, regardless of the scenario. Nurses need as extensive a repertoire as possible to address the multitude of patient responses that can occur in the course of our interaction with them.

In the scenario I just described, the physician decided to follow my nursing interventions because he had no biomedical interventions for the acute situation. The event prompted me to explore the differences between the biomedical and nursing models of patient care. I became interested in what nursing had to offer that biomedicine did not.

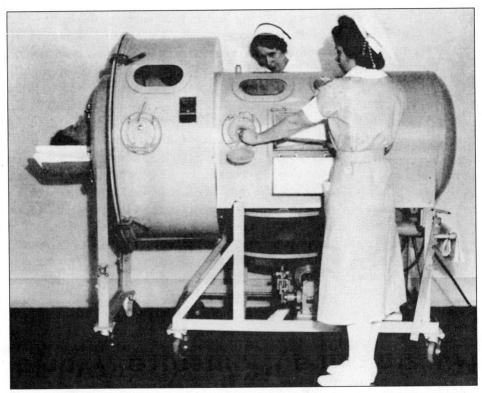

Nursing in a biomedical world, 1938 *(From Margaret Tracy,* Nursing: An Art and a Science. *St. Louis, MO: The C.V. Mosby Company, 1938. Used with permission.)*

Biomedicine

The world of biomedicine, or conventional medicine, is currently the dominant health culture in Western countries. I use the word *culture* because biomedicine involves a system of health beliefs and practices. Ethnographers such as Dr. Bonnie O'Connor have written about health belief systems. In her book, *Healing Traditions,* she states, "In the United States, as in any complex society, there is an encompassing 'official'—that is authorized and authoritative—culture, which coexists with any number of distinctive cultural subsets. The sanctioned practices, values, and institutions of the official culture are backed by considerable social, economic, and political power. Among these official values is the singular prestige accorded to science and its associated professions, and the sanction of formal education and academically legitimized research procedures (with a strong emphasis on scientific experimentation) as the primary—if not the sole—valid means to knowledge. Among the official institutions is a single authorized and legitimated system of health care" (O'Connor, 1995, p. 4). It is in this system, this culture, that professional nursing has developed. But just because nurses have worked side by side with physicians and supported the expansion of the biomedical model and culture does not mean that biomedicine represents the totality of nursing culture and nursing health beliefs.

Nurses have traditionally been involved in all aspects of the health of patients. They realize the importance of the patient's unique experience of health and health care. Nurses understand the human science of caring for patients in addition to the biological, cure-based science of the medical profession. Nurses have developed a professional culture in which the focus is caring, comfort, and the development of a healing relationship in which the patient is valued as a whole person.

The development of the biomedical system began with very different principles and understanding. It was based on a conception of the body as a machine and the theory of Descartes, who stressed the dualism between mind and body. "Cartesian dualism is clearly evident to this day in the conceptual distinction between 'disease' and 'illness,' referring to the objective evidence and the subjective experience, respectively, that characterizes contemporary western biomedicine" (Thorne, 1993, p. 1932).

Biomedicine has been defined further in the following way: "In the mid-1800's, the medical system we now refer to as biomedicine began to dominate the health care scene. Biomedicine was shaped by two important sets of observations made in the early 1800's: (1) specific organ entities—bacteria—were responsible for producing particular disease states and characteristic pathological damage, and (2) certain substances—antitoxins and vaccines—could improve an individual's ability to ward off the effects of these and other pathogens. As their conquests mounted, biomedical scientists came to believe that once they found the offending pathogen, metabolic error, or chemical imbalance, all afflictions—including many mental illnesses—would eventually yield to the appropriate vaccine, antibiotic, or chemical compound" (Dossey & Swyers, 1992, p. xxxviii). This statement reflects the foundations of biomedical practice, something nurses understand very well from education and experience. Biomedicine, with its principles of objectivism and positivism, does not define nursing nor does it define all health systems and health beliefs. Biomedicine as a health care system is in its infancy. Compare biomedical thought with Chinese or Native American health care beliefs and practices, which have existed for hundreds of years and are still active today, often existing side by side with biomedicine.

One reason many traditional or vernacular healing traditions still exist today is the limitations of biomedicine. The biomedical emphasis on objectivism, dualism (mind-body split), determinism, and the body as a machine has been found lacking in communities suffering from increasing numbers of stress-related disorders and complex, chronic illnesses. One physician writes of this concern, "This model [biomedicine] has served us well, but with the progressive urbanization of life accompanied by the industrial and technologic revolutions humankind has seen the development of new and very different adversities, which have resulted in the emergence of a uniquely new category of modern day ailments, particularly stress-related diseases, acute and chronic that are directly linked to personal attitudes and lifestyle. As a result, the limitations of a medical model that cannot effectively incorporate psychological, psychosocial or spiritual factors—factors that are at the source of these ailments—has become increasingly evident" (Dacher, 1995, p. 187). Dacher identifies stress-related illness and illness related to attitudes and lifestyle as areas of limitation for biomedicine. Nursing practice and theory commonly address lifestyle, life stressors, and attitudes. Yet it is only recently, perhaps with the development of nursing theory over the past twenty years or so, that the ability of nurses to work directly with such health conditions has been given greater emphasis.

In the past, nurses were educated in the biomedical belief system because much of nursing work was done primarily in hospitals where the biomedical system is the dominant philosophy and practice. Much nursing education has developed out of the need for nurses to be an integral part of supporting biomedical objectives. One example is antibiotic administration.

DISCOVERY OF ANTIBIOTICS

Antibiotics were considered miracle drugs. When antibiotics were discovered, the "answer" had been found to the question of how to destroy the germs causing certain illnesses. Nurses dutifully administered the prescribed medication to patients either by mouth or by injection. Many lives were saved, and nursing was part of the victory. I've given antibiotics many times. I've often wondered what nursing would be like without antibiotics. Most assuredly I would have witnessed more deaths than I have. But I've also seen problems with the use and subsequent overuse of the miracle cure, antibiotics.

I've worked on pediatric units where resistant strains of bacteria grew as a result of excessive antibiotic use. I've taken care of elderly patients with infections for which there was no antibiotic treatment because of antibiotic resistance. I myself, as a sixteen-year-old girl, having had antibiotics rarely as a young child, developed a chronic tonsillitis that was completely resistant to antibiotics and which ultimately lead to a tonsillectomy. Much has been written about the overprescription of antibiotics by physicians and the need to retrain physicians regarding the appropriate use of antibiotics. What have nurses been doing during this evolution in biomedical practice?

Nurses care for the patients with infections. Nurses administer the medicine, which represents new hope for a cure, a defeat of the "enemy" bacteria. Nurses hold the hands of, and comfort, the frustrated patients who are placed on countless rounds of antibiotics in hopes of killing the bacteria "causing" their illness, only to find that they still have the infection, along with a serious secondary systemic yeast infection and gastrointestinal problems resulting from chronic antibiotic use. Nurses have taken on the additional responsibility of providing the drugs prescribed by physicians. That responsibility has taken on new meaning as nurses find that they can be indicted for murder when mistakes in medication administration cause the untimely death of a patient. Such was the case in the United States in Colorado where nurses were indicted for the crime of murdering a baby because they were the administrators of a deadly dose of antibiotic. Authorities implied that the nurses alone were responsible for the death by indicting only the nurses. The physicians and pharmacists involved were not indicted. I sat in the courtroom as the nurses stood trial and watched history in the making. One nurse was acquitted at trial and two accepted plea bargains (Nursing Management, 1998).

Nurses have dutifully stood by biomedical practitioners in their quest for "the cure," both when victories have been won and when the "cure" has caused great suffering. For nurses, the experience with antibiotics has been a mixed bag. Some nurses have begun to question the decision made long ago by other nurses to give medications in the first place. In the late 1980s, the American Medical Association proposed implementing a new hospital position, medication technician. Perhaps it would be in nursing's best interest to let go of medication administration altogether, unless the nurse giving the medication is the nurse prescribing the medication, as in the case of a nurse practitioner. As nursing looks at whether to begin prescribing medications directly, we may be taking on another tremendous problem facing the medical profession, that of drug interactions. Nurses need to look at the whole picture and decide if the benefits of nurses prescribing or administering medications to patients outweigh the risks. It may seem a radical departure from conventional nursing practice to question the administration of medications. But these are the types of questions nurses continue to face in their ongoing interaction with the biomedical world.

Physicians are facing major challenges regarding the use of medications. A recent article in *Lancet* stated that *properly* prescribed drugs are now the fourth leading cause of death in the United States (Bonn, 1998). Will nurses be liable for these deaths simply because they administered the drugs?

In light of this information from *Lancet,* and the number of concerns around medication administration, the high-tech nature of pharmaceutical drugs may demand a specialist other than a professional nurse who already has a full day caring for patients without the added concern of pharmaceutical side effects and drug interactions. Is it important that we continue to identify nursing care with the administration of medications? Maybe yes, maybe no. What are the boundaries between nursing and biomedical care?

BOUNDARIES OF NURSING

No easy answers exist to this question or to the other questions surfacing as the identity of nursing undergoes significant change in the new millennium. What will the relationship between nursing and medicine be like? What nursing roles will be the same and what roles will change? Some nurses may not want to consider these issues.

I've certainly had many days when I did not want to deal with the changes in health care and nursing. In fact, I went to work in rural Montana thinking I was getting away from the chaotic issues of urban, high-tech health care. But I encountered the same issues in rural Montana as I had found in Los Angeles and Minneapolis. A shift is occurring in nursing, and it is felt wherever we practice. The minute we think we can just go to work and "do our job," we find that it is not that easy anymore. Every part of the health care system seems to be experiencing some level of chaos.

Chaos is derived from a Greek word meaning formless matter. Chaos is often perceived as complete confusion that is detrimental to life. But chaos can also be a tremendous opportunity for growth and change. "Modern science, however, teaches that chaos, or more specifically the edge of chaos, is a dynamic, holistic, and reciprocal process that drives change and creative reordering in systems. At the edge of chaos, where the turbulence exists, the system can either evolve to a higher level of complexity or collapse. The greatest degree of instability and resistance to change exists at this point. The current health care environment with its emphasis on the 'bottom line' is at this point. The system can tip in the direction of economics and deter human caring or create a new organizational pattern" (Ray et al., 1995, p. 48). The interaction and differentiation between nursing and biomedicine, along with the definition of nursing care, are major areas to be evaluated at the crossroads.

Lure of Technology

Western technology leads to powerful science and potent medicine. Its use in medical practice has improved our ability to define "problems" and design "cures." Technology is part of Western culture and is a way of life. In fact, many in society look to technology for answers in times of health crisis. Many nurses are part of technologically focused cultures. Nurses offer more than a problem-focused health experience and a cure. "Many practicing nurses have been educated in hospital schools of nursing. Nurses have been programmed to think that good care delivery is technologically driven, institutionally based, and oriented around the diagnosis and treatment of acute illness. . . . In the old days, nurses made the system work, around the clock, after the lights were dimmed, and the administrators, bookkeepers, and doctors had gone home" (Donley, 1996, pp. 329–330). Nurses know that their unique service to patients can exist even though it may only seem to come out in quiet when they alone stand with a patient. It is easy for the subtleties of nursing practice to be overpowered by biomedicine.

The medical practice model has clearly emphasized the development and use of technology as the gold standard for what constitutes modern medicine. Technology has been defined as "modalities and instrumentalities that greatly extend the power of human action, sensation, or thought in ways that are independent of the particular user" (Cassell, 1993, p. 32). Many technological advances in health care have improved health and reduced costs.

For example, the polio vaccine has saved many lives. When I was a school health nurse in Minnesota, I had a colleague who was a lieutenant colonel in the army. I substituted for her when she went to South America to administer polio vaccines to the people of a small country where vaccines were difficult to get and many were still dying from polio. When she returned, she told me that she gave vaccines all day long for days straight because the lines were so long. Death due to polio is virtually unheard of in the United States, so it is easy to forget that medical technology has often reduced mortality and had great benefit to society.

Technology has also proved disastrous at times. For example, the drugs diethylstilbestrol (DES®), fenfluramine-phentermine (Fen-phen®), and now Viagra® have harmed some people. Many babies never received the benefits of breast-feeding because the love of technology told us that formulas created by laboratory scientists must be better than mother's milk. Now we realize that mother's milk is the best food for newborns and science cannot replicate it. New is not synonymous with improved.

Even with these disastrous events, society and health care providers still look to technology for answers, hope, and promise. Technology is seductive. "Patients, their families and health care providers have become enticed by the magic and power of technology as it helps to win the battle over disease" (Erlen, 1994, p. 51). Nurses appreciate the intensity of a health crisis. Nurses are often at patients' sides as they experience pain, suffering, confusion, questioning, and fear when they become ill. Illness is not easy to witness, especially if a patient is experiencing extreme anguish. Nurses try to help patients in a way that empowers them when they feel they've lost control.

PERCEPTION OF POWER

When I studied the Roy adaptation model of nursing, we learned about the importance of the patient's need to feel empowered. As I learned ways to facilitate this, especially with children, I found that I became empowered also. Power has become synonymous with helping patients. In a technological, biomedical world, the importance of power and control is everywhere.

Eric Cassell writes, "It is our power that technology expands" (Cassell, 1993, p. 32). I recognize the importance of this statement as one of the reasons I went into nursing after being a teacher for some time. I felt a terrible sense of powerlessness as I watched my three-year-old student and her mother as they were struck by a van one sunny afternoon after leaving the schoolyard. I heard brakes screech and then a big thump as I turned to see my sweet little student get up from the pavement and look at her mother, unconscious, pale, and lying in a heap in the street. I was the first person on the scene and had no idea what to do for them. It was a terrible feeling. My common sense had me stop traffic and get other bystanders to call the emergency team. I could do nothing for the mother, so I held the child and comforted her. I will never forget that sense of powerlessness as long as I live. It is what led me to go on to become a first aid and CPR instructor for the American Red Cross in addition to becoming a registered nurse.

I have witnessed the same sense of powerlessness in nurse colleagues as well as in patients and their families. Although I have grown more comfortable with the fact that I may be unable to act in some situations, and that there are always new learning experiences, I have noticed that as a technologically oriented society, we are often not comfortable with the unknown or ambiguous. "Technology holds sway over medicine and its public because of its self-perpetuating character and its enhancement of power, as well as its capacity to induce wonder, root us in the immediate, remove ambiguity and increase certainty. Since this is not well understood, it is hardly surprising that technology, by itself inert and useless (although beckoning for attention through its inherent purposes), should be blamed for the troubles it brings. The real culprits are the doctors who use it, the public that loves it and the narrow knowledge on which it is based" (Cassell, 1993, p. 39).

Caring for people, especially when they are suffering, is often a complicated task. Some caregivers feel more confident caring for people when their environment, treatments, and assessment methods are organized and routine, even standardized. Most health care providers, especially in a litigious society such as the United States, prefer to remove as much ambiguity from the health care equation as possible. "Virtually all technology is marked by similarly unambiguous values. In fact, lack of ambiguity is essential to good medical science" (Cassell, 1993, p. 35). Although one goal of technology is to decrease ambiguity, is it realistic to presume it possible to achieve a practice free of ambiguity by increasing the use of technology? It seems more reasonable to think that a better goal when working in the human sciences might be to have greater tolerance and understanding of the nature of ambiguity.

Nurses are often more comfortable with the ambiguities of care because the foundation of their practice lies in developing a healing relationship with a patient and caring for the person. We listen to the patient and create a plan of care that is appropriate for the individual. We recognize the uniqueness of the individual's response to life challenges such as illness. As practitioners, we are adaptable. Nurses who demonstrate flexibility and tolerance for differences and ambiguities are often more experienced in their understanding of the human condition and the nature of a healing relationship.

The best training I got in tolerance of ambiguity and understanding differences was when I worked in rural health care. The little cabins we worked in were nothing like the hospitals I had worked in, where everything I needed, from equipment to phones to doctors and other colleagues, was accessible. This is not so in rural care. We often had to use what we had available for such things as pain management and triage. Working in a rural health office often felt like a "trial by fire," but through it all I discovered how resourceful my nurse colleagues and I were and how much I valued common sense as well as my education in biomedical and caring skills. Common sense becomes even more important with the expansion of technology.

Common sense is one aspect of the intuitive process of knowing. Losing common sense is a potential side effect of interaction with high technology. For example, I once worked with a nurse who had been working in the intensive care unit for a number of years. Once, when we were visiting a school together, she got unnerved when she did not know how to help a child who had a bloody nose. She could not even remember to offer the child a tissue. She felt that she had lost her common sense.

Although I have tremendous gratitude for the technological developments of the last few decades, I also realize that to allow technologies such as medical equipment and pharmaceutical drugs to continue to dictate nursing practice would be wrong. "It is fair to say that many patients believe that it is the test rather than the physician that makes the diagnosis, and the drug rather than the physician that effects the cure" (Cassell, 1993, p. 37). If nurses, in the struggle for power, assurance, and certainty, focus more and more on biomedical reductionism and technology, might patients someday think that it is the technology that does the "nursing" too? Will nursing care become associated only with the ability to keep machines running properly and give medications correctly? "Machines can seem so accurate, so right. They can make us forget who made them, and who designed them—with all the possibilities of human frailty and error—the programs that dictate their function. They make us forget the hands and minds behind their creation; they make us forget ourselves" (Reiser, 1984, p. 18).

Holism versus Reductionism

The biomedical world nurses practice in is based on the concept of "reductionism." Reductionism in medicine is the concept that all illness, including all of its cultural, social, physical, and emotional components, can be reduced, or explained by the biological problem. Hence the concept that the human body is like a machine. Scientists investigate diseases, and their findings become the oversimplified picture of an illness experienced by a patient. For instance, in infectious disease the focus of the interaction between patient and health care provider often becomes the identification and eradication of the germ involved. The disease becomes identified with the germ rather than the patient. Nurses have been part of the education of patients regarding their germs, diseases, and subsequent treatments. We often act as translators between physicians and patients, translating the language of the biomedical belief system of illness. But we also have our own beliefs about health, disease, and healing. It is important for nurses to remember that the biomedical belief in reductionism is relatively new and that it is just one of many health belief systems. Yet it is a belief system that has tremendous power in many countries.

For this reason, it is understandable how nurses became interested in and educated in this belief system and how it manifests in the choices physicians make regarding how they provide health care. Nurses, too, make choices about the interventions they provide to patients from their own belief system. Often, our values and beliefs drive our choices. Because nurses provide care from a different belief system, the care nurses provide is quite different than the care offered by those practicing from a biomedical perspective. There are some big philosophical differences between nursing and the biomedical belief system.

Dr. Beryla Branson Wolf, a nurse, did an extensive study of nursing identity and the relationship between the disciplines of nursing and medicine (1989). Dr. Wolf found that the values and beliefs of the nursing and medical professions are sometimes quite different. She found that nursing's core values are "persons as individuals and wholeness in life" and that the process by which nursing manifests its values is "caring." She found that medicine's core values are responsibility and human life and that the way medicine manifests its core values is "making a difference." Dr. Wolf also found that "medicine values the biological aspects of life more highly than does nursing and that nursing values the living aspects of life more highly than does medicine" (1989, p. iv). Hence the different focus in caring for others. Nurses want to know how a patient adapts to, or copes with, a particular health challenge. Physicians look primarily at the biological aspects thought to be causing the challenge.

This study shows clearly that both professions demonstrate caring and "make a difference in the lives of people." Nurses define the focus of their philosophy of caring as that of wholeness, balance, how to live, and how to create healing relationships. "Medicine demonstrates caring by making a difference, adding possibilities for life that would not exist without the medical perspective. Medicine adds life possibilities from without. Using caring as an epistemology and methodology, nursing enables persons to make existing and provided possibilities come into being and work within their lives" (Wolf, 1989). Nurses manifest their core values by "seeking to know the patient as he or she defines and manifests self. This type of knowing occurs within the nurse-patient relationship and is transcendent knowing in that it does not entail subject-object boundaries" (p. 288).

Nursing values the nurse-patient relationship, through which the nurse gets to know a patient's needs and develop a plan of care with the patient. Nurses do not value the identification of a patient's disease process and the ability to identify a biological malfunction. Nurses gain more information and gain a more solid understanding of patients and their needs when they have the "whole picture." This whole picture or holistic approach to working with patients is not reductionistic. The holistic approach is more appropriate for nursing. One approach is not better than the other, and nurses can certainly think in reductionistic terms, but ultimately, in creating a plan of care with a patient, we value and utilize our understanding and belief in a holistic process.

NURSES' HOLISTIC PROCESS

The holistic process begins with the assessment. Nurses are educated to begin assessment from the time they begin engaging with a patient. A nurse may walk into a patient's room, take one look at the patient and know that something is "wrong." Nurses are trained to see the "whole picture," and if that picture is not balanced, the nurse usually starts an assessment. The patient could be manifesting a mood change or be vomiting. There is no difference to the nurse between mind, body, and spirit behaviors. They are all parts of the human experience, and our assessment skills and interventions are capable of addressing the whole person. The people we care for have been called many things—patients, clients, guests, etc. But to nurses, they are people. Nurses practice holistic care with people because the focus is the whole person.

Although nurses' core values are about caring and the healing relationship with patients, I have often seen the pressures of the biomedical world—its biological values and technologies—interfere with the nursing process, nursing values, and tradition. In 1987, I began working on a pediatric intensive care unit for a large teaching hospital in the Midwest. While mentoring on the unit, I was made aware of a seven-year-old child who was there for monitoring, tests, and intravenous medications. The child was unable to communicate verbally because of developmental delays. The hospital was a teaching hospital for medical residents, so basic nursing functions such as starting IVs were not done by nurses, but rather by the residents.

This child was considered a real "problem patient" by the staff because they could not communicate with her and she kept pulling out her IV lines. The residents had ordered that the girl be restrained, and their plan was to sedate her after restarting her IV.

As I entered the child's room, I noticed the child's grandmother sitting in a chair in the corner. As I began my assessment of the child, who was writhing in the bed, I started a conversation with the grandmother. She told me that she was distraught by the thought of restraining and sedating the child. She confided in me that she thought her granddaughter was pulling out her lines because a diaper rash was making her uncomfortable. As I continued my assessment and removed the girl's diaper, I found that, indeed, this child had one of the worst diaper rashes I had ever seen.

My assessment told me that the diaper rash needed to be attended to immediately. I had worked in a large pediatric institution where an enterostomal nurses' concoction, called "butt paste," was used routinely for diaper rash with tremendous success. I convinced the residents to give it a try before resorting to sedation. Within an hour after the paste was applied, the child slept soundly, and the grandmother was showing tears of gratitude.

After this experience, I started to wonder what was happening in health care that physicians were missing opportunities to heal without drugs or procedures that have potential side effects. Were the residents not interested in finding the cause of the child's discomfort? Sedation, especially for a child who could not protest verbally, seemed like too easy an answer.

Many nurses work in a biomedical world much like the world I experienced on this unit. How can nurses maintain an identity as holistic practitioners in such a setting? The first step is to identify the biomedical health belief system in action, know what it is about, and how it manifests in patient care. Then, nurses will be aware of when our work, and our way of interacting with patients, lies outside the biomedical belief system. I believe that the little girl with the diaper rash needed a nurse as well as a doctor to provide her care. In this scenario, the residents were accepting of and grateful for my suggestion and experience. This is not always the case. Providing holistic patient care often means being a patient advocate in a world where the patient may be forgotten in the quest for the cure.

Conclusion

Nursing is at a crossroads. Since the 1980s, nurse theorists have laid a foundation on which we can build our identity as a profession in a bigger way. Now, as we begin the new millennium, we need to identify interventions—ways in which we demonstrate our core values of creating healing relationships and caring—that differentiate our care from the biomedical approach to patient care. Abundant opportunities exist for developing both old and new modalities through which nurses can demonstrate caring.

References

Bonn, D. (1998). Adverse drug reactions remain a major cause of death. *Lancet, 351,* 1183.

Cassell, E. J. (1993). The sorcerer's broom: Medicine's rampant technology. *Hastings Center Report, 23* (6), 32–39.

Dacher, E. S. (1995). A systems theory approach to an expanded medical model: A challenge for biomedicine. *The Journal of Alternative and Complementary Medicine, 1* (2), 187–196.

Donley, Sr. R. (1996). Nursing at the crossroads. *Nursing Economics, 14* (6), 325–331.

Dossey, L., & Swyers, J. (1992). Alternative medicine: Expanding medical horizons, A report to the National Institutes of Health on Alternative Medical Systems and Practices in the United States. Washington, DC: U.S. Government Printing Office, xxxviii–xlvii.

Erlen, J. (1994). Technology's seductive power. *Orthopedic Nursing, 13* (6), 50–52.

Nursing Management (1998). *Voices from Colorado, 29* (6): 52–53.

O'Connor, B.B. (1995). *Healing traditions: Alternative medicine and the health professions.* Philadelphia: University of Pennsylvania Press.

Ray, M., Didominic, V., Dittman, P., Hurst, P., Seaver, J., Sorbello, B., & Stankes-Ross, M. (1995). The edge of chaos. *Nursing Management, 26,* 48–49.

Reiser, S. (1984). *The machine at the bedside: Strategies for using technology in patient care.* Cambridge, England: Cambridge University Press.

Thorne, S. (1993). Health belief systems in perspective. *Journal of Advanced Nursing, 18,* 1931–1941.

Wolf, B. B. (1989). *Nursing identity: The nursing-medicine relationship.* Unpublished doctoral dissertation, University of Colorado, Denver.

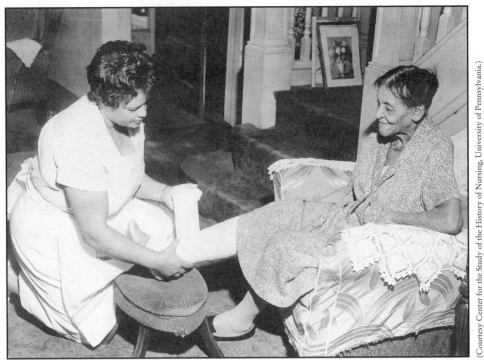

Hands-on care

Without tradition, art is a flock of sheep without a shepherd.

Without innovation, it is a corpse.

—WINSTON CHURCHILL

CHAPTER 2

Integrative Nursing:
Illusory, Idealistic, or Imperative?

Nurses enter the nursing profession for a variety of reasons. Whatever the motivations, people become nurses and go through years of education and clinical practice because, at some level of their being, they like to care for others. Caring is what nurses do, and it is who we are as professionals. From the time we begin learning about caring for people, we begin to develop a personal philosophy about what it means for us, personally and professionally, to take care of others.

One of Merriam-Webster's definitions of philosophy is "a theory underlying or regarding a sphere of activity or thought" (Merriam-Webster's Collegiate Dictionary, 1999). Over the years, nurses' philosophy of caring becomes more and more refined. What is frustrating for many nurses is that they learn the "ideal" of caring for patients when they are in school and the realities of practice never seem to measure up to that learned standard of care.

Nurses often talk about having to compromise their philosophy of nursing and their standard of care because of organizational goals and pressures of the day-to-day tasks they perform in a variety of settings. As nurses mature in their profession, and develop their own caring philosophy, they are often confronted with the seeming antagonism between what many call the "realities" of the "job" of nursing and the "ideals" of providing nursing care.

The obstacles to realizing the ideals for nursing care are not just the duties or tasks we perform. A qualitative study done by nurses examined the spiritual nursing interventions provided by mental health nurses (Tuck, Pullen, & Lynn, 1997). In this qualitative study, fifty mental health nurses were asked to complete three open-ended interrogative statements in addition to filling out the Spiritual Perspective Scale, a demographic questionnaire. The first statement asked the nurses to describe the ideal spiritual interventions with patients. One of the findings of the study was quite interesting. The investigators found that "mental health nurses perceive themselves as having a high level of spirituality. . . . They value spiritual interventions and think it is a part of care but few report instances of actually intervening" (p. 362). Some examples of the spiritual care mentioned in the study were doing a spiritual assessment, providing emotional support, listening, showing respect for religious beliefs, and helping patients connect with internal and external belief systems. The authors of the study suggest that possible reasons for the nurses not performing interventions they personally value are that they may need education in providing spiritual interventions, they may have felt some level of discomfort in providing spiritual interventions to patients, they may have identified spirituality too closely with religion, or they were uncomfortable with religious issues. Whatever the reasons, the nurses did not give the kind of patient service they valued. What is also interesting about another study by Sodestrom and Martinson (1987) is that about half of the clients interviewed in the study depended on the nurse for spiritual guidance. How often do patients expect and even depend on nurses to provide some type of care and yet not receive it even though nurses may have the same expectation?

The obstacles to providing care to our patients come from within ourselves and within our profession, as well as from the tasks, schedules, and requirements placed upon us from administrators and health care institutions. As nurses look to the future of nursing practice in the new millennium, and within a changing model of health care, now is the time for us to make our philosophies of caregiving known. Nursing philosophy of health care needs to be represented in the "big picture" of the future of health care. Jean Watson, nurse theorist and educator writes, "When approaching a crossroads between centuries, worldviews, paradigms, and research traditions, new questions must be asked and new challenges faced. . . . We have often allowed biomedical knowledge alone to define for us ethical and moral issues of being a scientist or a medical professional, and even what it means to be human" (Watson, 1995, p. 64).

Biomedicine has meant a great deal to many people who have seen their loved ones healed of diseases that were once deadly. The surgical techniques, pharmaceuticals, research, and technology of biomedicine have been a boon to the industrialized West. But there are growing concerns about the inability of biomedicine to deal expertly with stress-related illness, infection, chronic illnesses such as cancer and heart disease, and psychiatric illness, to name just a few.

In 1977, Engel created a new medical model to address some of these concerns. He identified some of the problems in biomedicine as "such undesirable practices as unnecessary hospitalization, overuse of drugs, excessive surgery and inappropriate use of diagnostic tests" (Engel, 1977, p. 134). Of course, managed care emerged later to supposedly put an end to many of these problems.

Engel also wrote of growing consumer concerns over the shortcomings of biomedicine as well. "There is a growing uneasiness among the public . . . that health needs are not being met and that biomedical research is not having a sufficient impact in human terms. Physicians lack interest and understanding, are preoccupied with procedures, and are insensitive to the personal problems of patients and their families. Medical institutions are seen as cold and impersonal" (Engel, 1977, p. 129). Engel's new model attempted to broaden the medical model to include psychosocial issues as well. Some medical practitioners, primarily family medicine practitioners, have incorporated the psychosocial needs of patients into their practice.

Nurses have always focused on the psychosocial needs of patients because, by the very nature of their work, they have always practiced holistically. With all the concerns of biomedicine, it would seem impractical for nurses to continue to uphold the biomedical model or belief system as the gold standard when it is clear that biomedicine is in the throes of many challenges, and that health care consumers are unhappy with the continued emphasis on the biomedical model. It seems imperative that nurses begin to claim the worthiness of their own beliefs, paradigms, philosophies, and theories of health, healing, and caring. "For too many years we have been delegated practices; we have been the eyes, ears, and hands of other professionals when it has been expedient or convenient. Nursing practice is nursing practice because it is grounded in nursing knowledge. This is an important point during this time of health care reform when nurses may be co-opted to provide labor for a system that is parallel to and less expensive than the current one, but is substantively no different from it. Our practice provides a unique and valuable service to society and we need to engage in it full-time" (Smith, 1994, p. 6). There is so much that nursing has to offer.

In *Notes on Nursing,* Florence Nightingale emphasized the necessity of an expanding body of knowledge distinct from medical knowledge. Nightingale believed that "'Nursing should be a search for truth. It should be the discovery of God's laws of healing and their proper application.' Physical healing for Nightingale is a natural process regulated by law. She believed that nursing is providing an environment which facilitates, rather than disturbs, the natural healing process, through the use of fresh air, sunlight, warmth, quiet, and cleanliness. The basic needs of the sick, she insisted, derive from natural laws and thus are timeless and universal" (Macrae, 1995, p. 9).

Nurses are aware of these natural laws because they see the laws play out before their eyes every day in the lives of their patients and in their healing relationships with patients. Nurses who seek further discovery of natural law become more consciously aware of the importance of their everyday tasks to their patients and to their own personal well-being as nurse-healers. The remainder of this book discusses the many ways nurses demonstrate caring through various modalities and the healing relationships that are formed as a result of that caring process. This focus on building healing relationships, and the creative ways of demonstrating care, leads nurses toward an exploration of the numerous ways to integrate their caring and biomedical skills in a practice I call integrative nursing.

Integrative Nursing Defined

Integrative nursing is the creation of evolving, healing relationships with patients. The nurse observes the patient's needs for greater harmony and balance in their life and then addresses those needs by offering care that is a holistic blend of biomedical and caring modalities. The integrative nurse finds creative ways to integrate or harmonize his skills in the service of others. To integrate also means to embody. The integrative nurse demonstrates the science and art of nursing out of a deep sense of having embodied, or having made a genuine part of their being, their own personal identity as a professional nurse.

The guiding principles of the practice of integrative nursing are balance and homeostasis, keen observation and holism, and the use of biomedical and caring skills in a creative way that addresses the individual needs of patients (see Figure 2–1).

Each integrative nurse works in a collaborative relationship with the patient as well as with other health care providers. The reason for the emphasis on collaboration is the understanding of the development of the healing relationship as foundational to nursing practice. The healing relationship model for integrative nursing practice depicted here will be discussed in more detail in Chapter 12. It is presented here so that, as the components of integrative nursing are discussed, you might begin

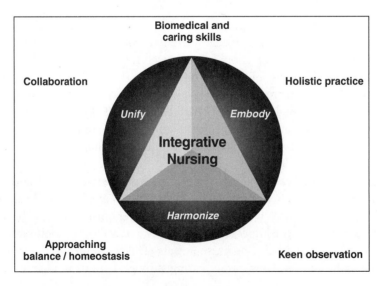

FIGURE 2–1

Integrative Nursing

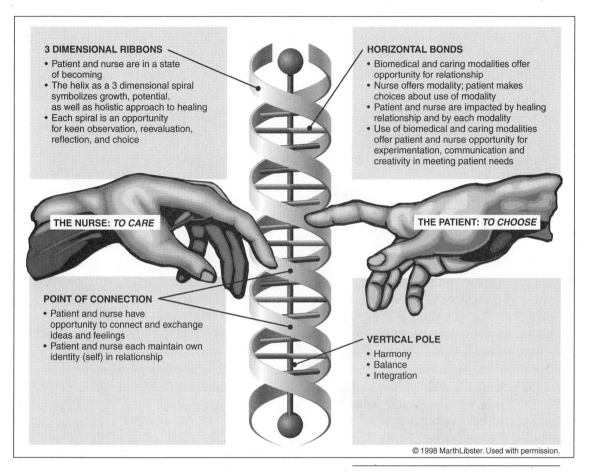

3 DIMENSIONAL RIBBONS
- Patient and nurse are in a state of becoming
- The helix as a 3 dimensional spiral symbolizes growth, potential, as well as holistic approach to healing
- Each spiral is an opportunity for keen observation, reevaluation, reflection, and choice

HORIZONTAL BONDS
- Biomedical and caring modalities offer opportunity for relationship
- Nurse offers modality; patient makes choices about use of modality
- Patient and nurse are impacted by healing relationship and by each modality
- Use of biomedical and caring modalities offer patient and nurse opportunity for experimentation, communication and creativity in meeting patient needs

THE NURSE: *TO CARE*

THE PATIENT: *TO CHOOSE*

POINT OF CONNECTION
- Patient and nurse have opportunity to connect and exchange ideas and feelings
- Patient and nurse each maintain own identity (self) in relationship

VERTICAL POLE
- Harmony
- Balance
- Integration

© 1998 MarthLibster. Used with permission.

FIGURE 2–2

Healing relationship model for integrative nursing practice

to see how integrative nursing practice is related to the creation of healing relationships (see Figure 2–2). Creating and participating in healing relationships can be a dynamic, energizing experience. This experience, if depicted as a geometric form, could be drawn as a helix or a three-dimensional spiral (see Figure 2–3). The spiraling movement of this shape represents continuation, momentum, and potential. The helix spiral represents the creation of healing relationships as an ongoing process that can gain momentum. The three-dimensional nature of the helix represents the multi-dimensionality of the process of building a healing relationship. Like the carving movement of a spiraling helix, healing relationships are "carved" out by the people involved. Patients facing challenging health conditions must carve out a new way of being, and the nurse supports the process. The nurse interacts with the patient's helical path.

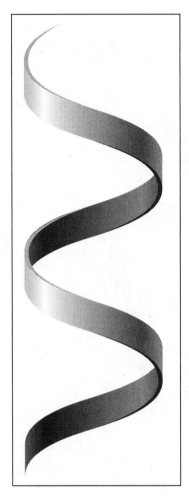

FIGURE 2-3
Single helix

The double helix is a metaphor for the process of creating healing relationships in integrative nursing practice. Both the nurse and the patient are active participants in a healing relationship. They are each represented by one ribbon or helix. Each person in a healing relationship has her own path as represented in the separateness of the ribbons, but these paths overlap, as shown in Figure 2–2, as points of connection. These points of connection represent times when the nurse and patient share ideas and feelings. The horizontal bonds between the helices represent the relationship itself. The bonds are formed when the nurse offers care to the patient and the patient chooses to accept. In the healing relationship, both the nurse and the patient can receive healing. As a vertical pole supports the action of the double helix, so too is the action of the healing relationship supported by the focus on the goals of greater harmony, integration, and balance.

BALANCE AND HOMEOSTASIS

Pretend that you are a patient for a moment. Pretend that you have pain, excruciating pain. Perhaps your head is so painful and throbbing that you begin pulling at your hair. You have taken the pain medication, but it's going to take thirty minutes to start working, if it works at all. You know that the medication doesn't always work because the headaches have happened before. The pain continues. In walks a friend who offers to massage your back and feet and puts a warm water bottle behind your neck. She stays with you, gently coaxing you to breathe and not fight the pain. She draws your attention away from the head pain by causing some tenderness on your feet with her deep massage strokes. Before you know it, the pain is easing, the medicine is taking effect, your breathing is easy. You fall fast asleep.

Nurses often find themselves in the position of being the one to care for someone experiencing serious physical, emotional, or spiritual pain or discomfort. Often, we offer our patients the best of biomedicine—drugs. We are also in the position of carrying out the orders for high-tech treatments that ultimately lead to cures for various illnesses. This is what we learn from biomedicine. This is our established role in the world of biomedicine. But what about all the other things we do with patients to help them adapt, cope, and live with their diseases? Let's go back to the headache scenario. How would you feel if the only choice you had was to take a pain reliever for the headache and lie in bed waiting for the drug to take effect, praying that it would indeed take effect?

Integrative nursing is the professional practice of caregiving in which the nurse combines biomedical knowledge and techniques with caring modalities in a holistic way when entering a healing relationship with patients. Many nurse theorists have envisioned nursing as the synchrony of our biomedical knowledge with our caring practices. For example, Hildegarde Peplau suggests a "constructive blend . . . that would enhance nursing practice defined as nursing science applied within a highly sophisticated compassionate art" (Peplau, 1988, p. 14). Often, nursing literature defines the art of nursing by the ways we care for others. Nurses demonstrate compassion, empathy, and caring through acts of genuine kindness such as getting someone a glass of cool water when they are thirsty, or changing the soiled bed of an elderly hospice patient. Everything we do is about kindness. Everything we do is about helping people realize what it means for them to be "ill" and what it means for them to feel "well." We help people realize their physical, emotional, and spiritual strengths and limitations. And we often do a lot of our work attending to the needs of others in a moment of crisis, a healing crisis.

Crises in life can be big or small. Regardless of the extent of the crises, they are always important to the persons involved and they always demand the ability to change and/or adapt. Health crises call a patient and a caregiver's attention to some imbalance in the life of the patient. Understanding the need for restoration of balance or equilibrium by assisting the body's natural quest for homeostasis is the first component in the practice of integrative nursing.

There is often a fine line between helping the body and interfering with the body and its ability to heal and restore balance. For example, putting a baby in a warm bath can be a very caring and soothing thing to do for a baby with a tummy upset. But leaving the baby in the water until the water turns cold is no longer caring. Nurses can learn from patients themselves what is needed to restore their own sense of balance and harmony both within themselves and with their environment.

Balance is best achieved when nurses act in ways that enable the best use of technologies for a patient. They must be aware that, "The goal is not to use as much technology as possible, but rather to use technology skillfully to work toward the goals established among the patient, family, and health professionals" (Erlen, 1994, p. 52). The balanced use of technology with patients is essential to respectful nursing care. Nurses demonstrate respect for patients when they support a patient's right to choose and utilize any modality for healing, whether it is chemotherapy or the laying on of hands. Not all patients desire many choices or are able to choose, but those who wish to be the decision makers in their own health care are often better able to adapt to their health situation or concern when given the opportunity to be involved.

"The ancient Greeks believed that one was to live with and adapt to the world in which one lived rather than to conquer it" (Erlen, 1994, p. 51). The ability of a person to adapt involves a change in her internal environment. To understand these internal changes one must understand homeostasis and balance. The term *homeostasis* is derived from two Greek words, *homeo* meaning staying the same and *stasis* meaning standing still.

The human body is expert at the process of adaptation in an attempt to maintain balance and homeostasis. Regulation of body temperature, blood glucose, and pH balance are all examples of the body's ability to maintain homeostasis. Homeostasis is essential to life, for the survival of cells and bodily systems. "Homeostasis is regulated in the short term by the nervous system and in the longer term by the endocrine system. The maintenance of homeostasis, on the other hand, is achieved by the participation, cooperation and interdependency of all the systems of the body" (Rinomhota & Cooper, 1996, p. 1102). Homeostasis is a holistic process that is not 100 percent infallible. Many nurses question whether *homeostasis* is the correct word to use to define the body's process of seeking harmony and balance. It is questionable that the body ever actually remains the same or stands still. For this reason some nurses prefer to use the concept of balance or harmony as opposed to homeostasis. Aging is an example of the shortcomings of the use of the word homeostasis.

Nurses are aware that as people get older their ability to adapt to external stimuli is more of a challenge. An older patient taking longer to bounce back from illness is an example of the slowing down of the body's ability to return to homeostasis. It is rare that the body stays the same or stands still in time and space. The biomedical term *homeostasis* is relative to the actual human processes observed in nursing practice. Patients go through many adaptive processes, both internal and external, in order to maintain a sense of harmony and balance as they experience changes throughout life. This adaptive process is dynamic and is not only observed by the nurse, but is also influenced by the nurse who is part of the patient's environment.

Balance and homeostasis refer to all the body's internal feedback loops for restoring and maintaining harmony. This includes emotional balance as well as physiological balance. Newer research in the area of psychoneuroimmunology by scientists such as Dr. Candice Pert is exploring, on the cellular level, the ability of emotions and cells of the body to "talk" to each other (Pert, 1997). We are whole beings in which the sum of the parts is much greater than the whole, probably much more wonderful than we know. But we can, if we choose to, wonder about, hope for, and imagine a health state, a harmonious state, with our patients that exemplifies the uniqueness of their feelings and becoming aware of a greater sense of wholeness and happiness. As nurses, we hold a belief in, and the vision of, our patients' wholeness and happiness. As long as we attend only to the biomedical reductionistic belief system in which the emphasis is to look scientifically at the parts of the human, we miss the opportunity to explore the possibilities for greater understanding of what health is about from the standpoint of the *interaction* of parts (spirit, mind, and body), the inner workings of the ways humans are able to achieve balance and harmony as represented in research by scientists such as Dr. Pert.

Dr. Pert gives the example in her book, *Molecules of Emotion,* of a patient's conscious effort to harness the body's homeostatic processes. She writes, "Conscious breathing, the technique employed by the yogi and the woman in labor, is extremely powerful. There is a wealth of data showing that changes in the rate and depth of breathing produce changes in the quality and kind of peptides that are released from the brain stem. And vice versa! By bringing this process into consciousness and doing something to alter it—either holding your breath or breathing extra fast—you cause the peptides to diffuse rapidly throughout the cerebro-spinal fluid, in an attempt to restore homeostasis, the body's feedback mechanism for restoring and maintaining balance. And since many of these peptides are endorphins, the body's natural opiates, as well as other kinds of pain-relieving substances, you soon achieve a diminution of your pain. So it is no wonder that so many modalities, both ancient and New Age, have discovered the power of controlled breathing" (Pert, 1997, pp. 186–187). For years, labor and delivery nurses have encouraged women in labor to breathe. It's so simple, and yet so complex, when a scientist delves into the happenings in the body on a cellular level. And how much time does it take to help a person to breathe when she is in pain?

Sometimes the most elusive interventions in nursing are the simplest. Perhaps nurses feel that the things they do, like reminding a patient to do some deep breathing, are too simple, even menial. We know from the Pert research that breathing interventions are critical to pain management, not to mention all the other bodily processes that purposeful deep breathing assists.

There are many seemingly menial tasks nurses engage in that are vital to the assistance of human life in restoring balance or homeostasis. Suzanne Gordon writes, "At one moment a nurse may be involved in a sophisticated clinical procedure that demands expert judgement and advanced training in the latest technology. The next moment she may do what many people consider trivial or menial work, such as emptying a bedpan, giving a spongebath, administering medication or feeding or walking a patient. It is only in watching nurses weave the tapestry of care that we grasp its integrity and its meaning for a society that too easily forgets the value of things that are beyond price" (1997, p. 88).

The basic hands-on bedside care the nursing profession has provided to the public for centuries is essential. The "menial" tasks, when done with the same effort, intention, and attention as the more demanding technological tasks will command the same respect and recognition. It is up to nurses to make it so.

For example, when I was a nursing student working as a nursing assistant in a hospital in an affluent area of Los Angeles, I had a male patient actually say to me, "You really enjoy emptying my bedpan, don't you?" At first, I was a little flustered that he could tell and I thought, "He probably thinks I'm weird." But I responded, "And I like making your bed, too, because it helps you feel comfortable, right?" He agreed with a smile. From that day on I made up my mind that I had to find a way to find importance in everything in my practice. Why perform high-tech care or back rubs if it means nothing to my patients or to me? In fact, I had to know what is important to patients when they are being cared for. I found out that not everyone wants the high-tech "cure," but everyone wants the bedpan emptied. Not everyone wants a back rub, but everyone expects to be treated with dignity and courtesy. I found out that many people use complementary therapies in addition to seeing their regular doctors. And, I've learned that people have their own caring needs and perceptions of what is caring behavior and which caring behaviors help them find greater balance and harmony in life. I learned this through observation.

OBSERVATION AND HOLISTIC CARE

Observation and holistic care is the second component of integrative nursing. Florence Nightingale said, "If you cannot get into the habit of observation one way or other, you had better give up being a nurse, for it's not your calling, however kind and anxious you may be" (Nightingale, 1969, p. 94). Nightingale believed that the purpose of observation was to increase health and comfort. She gives the example of attendants on a case who "knew perfectly well that the patient could not get well in such an air, in such a room, or under certain circumstances, yet have gone on dosing him with medicine, and making no effort to remove the poison from him, or him from the poison they knew was killing him" (p. 104). Often the basic tasks that are forgotten or delegated to assistants and unlicensed providers become the forgotten, seemingly meaningless, menial observations. But as Nightingale so eloquently describes in her book, it is the nurse's role to observe changes in the patient's behavior, abilities, and needs and to respond accordingly by changing the plan of care.

This means that patients must be cared for as individuals with unique health care needs. There is no cookbook approach to nursing care. No two patients with headaches are alike. One may have a headache because he drank too much the night before and his head pain may be throbbing all over his entire head. Another person may have a headache because she is experiencing extreme stress related to a difficult separation from a spouse. Her headache is in the back of her head and down to her shoulders. The woman might say that a warm bath, deep breathing, and a cup of hot tea will relieve her headache. The man might want to be left alone with a couple of pain pills to sleep in a dark room. There are numerous ways people choose to deal with their health concerns.

In integrative nursing practice, nurses demonstrate caring by being observers of what "works" for patients and what makes them happy. We provide information about choices the patient has for dealing with an imbalance. And we respect the patient's choice.

Astute nursing observation is also essential to developing a healing relationship with a patient and being prepared to provide holistic care. I found that I was more observant as a nurse after my training in traditional Chinese herbal medicine. In Chinese medicine, every detail the patient tells of his health concerns is important, including a painful toenail or a twitching eyelid. We learned how to interview a patient so that the patient would speak of these details. My experience is that patients, when asked how they are feeling, will quote their doctors' diagnoses and test results rather than discuss the intimate details of how they are feeling in body, mind, and spirit.

We also learned to perform pulse and tongue diagnosis and to add our observations to the patient profile for evaluation. I equate this in-depth observation process to the painting of a picture. A practitioner paints a picture of the patient from her observations and her descriptions of what is going on with the patient. It takes time sometimes for the picture to be completed, because the details of the picture must be revealed by the patient and observed by the nurse. This process implies a relationship between the observer and the observed. In the healing relationship, the nurse is interested in the lived experience of the patient. These experiences are what "paint the picture" of the patient as a unique *person,* as well as a patient.

"Nurses have shifted their attention towards their 'relationships' with patients" and in the holistic model of nursing care "the 'lived experience' of illness and health are crucial components of a model that locate disease only as one part of a complex matrix" (May & Fleming, 1997, p. 1096). Integrative nursing practice includes the essential component of astute observation so that each patient is treated as a unique human being with unique needs. This is the foundation for holistic care and thus integrative nursing practice.

The concept of holism is integral to most nursing theory and practice. Practicing holistically means that the nurse observes, assesses, and interacts with the whole patient. Some nurses pursue certification as "holistic nurses" in which their education is specialized. Holism, in reference to nursing practice, when used here, refers to its more general, historical meaning of caring for the physical, emotional, psychological, social, and spiritual needs of the patient. Although integrative nursing practice includes the concept of holism, a nurse who practices holistically does not necessarily practice integratively. Nurses who address the holistic needs of patients may or may not have as their goal to help the patient achieve greater balance. They may not have explored the practice of integrating biomedical and caring skills.

INTEGRATING BIOMEDICAL SKILLS AND CARING MODALITIES

The third foundational component of integrative nursing is the integration of biomedical skills and knowledge with caring modalities. This process is a creative one in which the nurse helps the patient identify the options for care. These options are not limited to biomedical interventions, but include the patient's requests, suggestions, and creative ideas about how they would like to deal with an illness or health concern. The nurse can also share options from her own unique knowledge base regarding comfort measures and caring modalities.

Timing and discernment are important in developing an integrated care plan with a patient. Biomedical understanding of disease progression and perceived prognosis can be helpful in determining timelines for treatments. Nurses need to be educated in communication skills that enable them to identify the emotional and spiritual needs of their patients as well as their physical needs. The nurse's discernment skills are critical for identifying the appropriateness of the intervention for a particular patient at a particular time. For example, it is not a wise plan for a woman who may be pregnant to have a deep abdominal shiatsu massage. Another example is the timing of medical procedures for hospitalized patients. Patients' sleep cycles are often disturbed by health care team members who need to do their work in a timely fashion, sometimes without regard to the needs of the patient. Many children's hospitals have proven that a health care team can listen to the needs of the patient and respect the healing processes of each patient. For example, in one children's hospital where I worked, all staff needing to perform a procedure went to the primary nurse first to ask when would be the best time to see the patient.

As discussed in Chapter 1, the technology and research of the biomedical world offer a strength and authority that can comfort patients when they feel weakened by their fears and anxieties about changes in their state of health. But technology and research can also hinder the healing process. Nurses are in the best possible position to help patients make decisions about the care they receive. They are also coordinators of care and are in the perfect position to advocate for the emotional and spiritual needs, as well as the physical needs, of the patient. Often, nurses know that the physical needs of the patients have to wait while the patient has a good cry or talks with a chaplain or family member. When health providers dehumanize a patient or treat him like a "body in the bed," or a "machine to be fixed," they potentially create a situation where a power struggle can occur between patient and caregiver. Patient care can become an issue of "patient compliance" or our will versus their will rather than caring for an individual with special needs. Some health care providers, including nurses, still seek patient compliance.

Using the term *compliance* with patients is inherently demeaning. After all, it is their body and their choice. Integrative nursing is not about making demands on patients that they do or do not comply with. Integrative nursing is not about power struggle. Power is a major part of the biomedical paradigm—power over the disease, power over the patient. Integrative nursing is about respectful, healing relationships. If power remains the primary issue in health care, then patients will always win, because their health care is their choice, not ours.

Often it is said that a "difficult" patient is one who questions the nurses' actions. Having worked in pediatrics, I know of no other kind of patient or family member. The concept of the difficult patient or difficult family member who questions the nurse can be reframed as a thoughtful, curious person who is interested in taking an active role in the healing process. I have found that I spend less energy with patients by taking a moment to answer their questions with my full attention to their concerns. Otherwise you end up spending lots of time dealing with their unresolved fears and concerns which tend to build up over time. In fact, I have often been proactive and have asked parents and patients about their questions to let them know that I am open to their concerns.

There are multiple benefits for nurses who, in a holistic way, explain the benefits and risks of interventions to patients, tell patients or family members what they are doing when they enter a patient's room, and request consent with each intervention. This type of communication demonstrates respect for the patient's rights, it demonstrates that the patient has a choice each moment they are being cared for, and it ultimately frees the nurse of the burden of becoming all-knowing. The nurse and the patient can then develop a relationship, a relationship of trust from which both can gain confidence, strength, and healing. "Focusing on the patient and respecting the patient's lifeplan are ways that the nurse demonstrates caring" (Erlen, 1994, p. 52). Practitioners and patients alike often seek opportunities for health and healing experiences that include individualized patient-centered care. Because of the growing depersonalization of care in the larger health care institutions, many patients seek health care from the complementary therapy practitioners who usually provide more personalized attention.

A Beginning Look at Complementary Therapies

In the United States, physicians such as Andrew Weil and James Gordon have been using the term *integrative medicine* to define the practice of medicine that incorporates both biomedicine and what the United States National Institutes of Health has called complementary and alternative medicine (CAM). The International Conference on Integrative Medicine web site defines integrative medicine as "spanning the biases of disciplines and cultures, taking a systems approach to the treatment of the patient as well as the physical disorder. It stresses prevention, self-care and establishing healing partnerships. Practitioners in every field are beginning to integrate allopathic (biomedical), behavioral medicine and alternative practices into their treatment protocols" (International Conference on Integrative Medicine, 1999).

With the development of integrative models of care in many disciplines, including medicine and nursing, perhaps a "common ground" will emerge. The integrative philosophies of nursing and medicine may help to create more unity and synergy between the two professions. As discussed in Chapter 1, there may always be some philosophical differences between how integrative nursing and medicine are practiced based upon our different core values. I saw these differences while working in an integrative medicine clinic for five years.

Two physicians, one specializing in emergency medicine and one in internal medicine, were the directors of the clinic. I joined the practice after hearing that, in addition to allopathic medicine that included drugs, surgery, and radiology, and standard outpatient nursing care, the clinic offered complementary therapies including chiropractic care, massage therapy, reflexology, colonic therapy, nutritional therapy, macrobiotic diet counseling, medical herbal medicine, jin-shin-jyutsu, and Chinese medicine, to name a few.

I wore many hats in this practice. I was the coordinator of the medicinal herb program. We grew over 100 herbs, harvested and wildcrafted the herbs, processed them and made our own teas, oils, and salves. I also practiced as a clinical herbalist, reflexologist, and jin-shin practitioner. I had education and experience in these three areas prior to joining the group. I also developed protocols for the use of the Electro-acuscope™ and Myopulse™, two machines the practice had acquired. We used the machines primarily for pain management, especially low back and joint/muscle pain.

Although we offered many CAM and allopathic/biomedical treatments and services in this practice, the nurses were only practicing the beginnings of what I have defined as integrative nursing. In general, the practice used a biomedical, problem-focused approach to care, rather than a holistic approach. Collaboration and communication was often difficult or nonexistent. Although both complementary therapies and biomedicine were offered to patients, they were not offered in an integrative approach. The patient was usually offered only those modalities provided by the practitioner she was seeing. There was no coordinator of care. The physicians' concept of integrative medicine was very different from my concept of integrative nursing. It was not enough for me that I was using complementary therapies in practice. In my practice I also focused on the development of a collaborative relationship with the patient and facilitated communication among health providers on behalf of the patient. Patients often get overwhelmed by the numerous therapies suggested by their practitioners. As a nurse, I have often been in the role of helping patients make the decisions as to what therapies are appropriate for them by helping them gather more information from their practitioners and other sources. My goal is to help a patient make a clear, conscious, and informed choice about her health care whether it includes a complementary therapy or not.

The medical model of valuing a cure and saving a life seems to foster a sense of urgency in the physicians I have worked with, which then manifests as doing "everything they can" for the patient, i.e., using so many therapies at once that the patient and practitioner can no longer observe which therapies, if any, actually help the patient. The numerous healing modalities often become a stumbling block in the patient's healing process. Also, my experience with the medical model of integrative medicine showed me that many physicians superimpose the biomedical belief system over the complementary therapies they are using and often find that the therapy is ineffective. This happened with herbal medicines. The physicians I worked with often prescribed herbs that they had perhaps read a little bit about as they would when prescribing a drug. For example, when I started at the clinic, every patient received a capsule of goldenseal and echinacea when coming down with a cold. There was no discovery of the appropriateness of these herbs for the individual. Nurses followed the protocol that anyone with cold symptoms should be given these herbs. This particular practice is not healthy for patients or plant populations. This was just one example of how the philosophy and focus of the group was more about the biomedical or allopathic and CAM therapies and treatments themselves than about a collaborative, integrative philosophy of patient care in which the focus is balance or homeostasis, holistic practice, observation of patient need, and the integration of conventional biomedical and complementary modalities.

"Conventional medical practice can benefit from the inclusion of some CAM practices. However, not all CAM practices are appropriate to medicine, medical research is not well suited to all CAM practices, and the growing executive authority of physicians in CAM is unjust given the role of others—from nurses to herbalists to religious healers—in CAM development" (Hufford, 1997, p. 81). Because nurses are taught to collaborate with patients and to individualize each care plan, they are ideally positioned to work with complementary therapies. Nurses, as trusted members of society, are well positioned to take an active role in the exploration of the integration of complementary therapies into mainstream health care. The integration of complementary therapies with biomedical skills is the same issue nurses face each day when they make decisions about how to integrate caring and biomedical skills. "Nurses are in a position to act as 'bridges' for providers in the health care system to understand why patients use alternative healing as well as to add legitimacy to the use of alternative healing modalities" (Engebretson, 1996, p. 99). Nurses, because of their holistic worldview, readily understand the value of alternative and complementary therapies, many of which are based upon the same holistic belief system as nursing practice. In fact, when the original list of CAM modalities was created by the National Center for Complementary and Alternative Medicine (NCCAM) at the National Institutes of

Health (NIH) in Washington DC, science-based nursing was on the list. From the biomedical perspective, nursing care is "alternative" to mainstream medicine.

CAM modalities in the United States have been defined in the oft-quoted article by Dr. David Eisenberg as, "Unconventional therapies not taught widely at U.S. medical schools or generally available at U.S. hospitals" (1993, p. 246). The Office of Alternative Medicine defines CAM as, "Covering a broad range of healing philosophies, approaches and therapies. It generally is defined as those treatments and health care practices not taught widely in medical schools, not generally used in hospitals, and not usually reimbursed by medical insurance companies" (Office of Alternative Medicine, 1998). The 1993 Eisenberg study and the results of a follow-up national survey in 1998 (Eisenberg, Davis, Ettner, et al.), showed that CAM modalities are very popular with the American public. The 1993 study showed that approximately one-third of Americans use some form of unconventional therapy as defined in the study, a trend that continued until 1997. The studies also showed that Americans were willing to spend $10.3 billion dollars out-of-pocket in 1990 and $12.2 billion in 1997 (up to $27 billion when adding expenditures for vitamins, herbs, classes, and books) for these unconventional therapies. Does this mean that Americans are enamored of the unconventional? Possibly, yes. It also means that many of the therapies defined by the biomedical world as "unconventional" are actually ancient therapies or based upon cultural healing practices used by various cultures for centuries. Some Americans may recognize these therapies as "old friends" while the newer high-tech modalities and drugs often remain suspect. "From childbirth to nutrition to emotional well-being, medicine has established claims to expertise and authority over many areas of life not viewed as medical in other cultures or at other times. Efforts at medical control are often intrusive and unwelcome" (Hufford, 1997, pp. 81, 82).

We know that many of the modalities now defined and labeled CAM are often health promotion and lifestyle practices. Nurses have encouraged patients for centuries to adopt healthy lifestyles and to find ways to achieve balance and wholeness. Massage and touch therapies, historically and currently used in nursing practice, are part of the healing practices of many cultures and have been for centuries. And although there may not be hundreds of clinical trials on the physiological benefits of massage or other common CAM therapies, in reality, a study conducted by the Office of Technology Assessment of the United States Congress suggested that, "only about 20 percent of modern medical remedies in common use have been scientifically proved to be effective; the rest have not been subjected to empirical trials of whether or not they work and, if so, how" (Brown, 1998, p. 90). For decades nurses have been taught massage or effleurage as a comfort measure if nothing else. In fact, many of the modalities listed by the NCCAM as complementary and alternative have historically been part of nursing practice. (See Appendix A.) The nursing profession's role in the reintegration of complementary therapies into mainstream health practices in the West is just beginning to be defined.

Conclusion

Many nurses have become interested in complementary therapies. Often those who want to practice complementary therapies leave the field of nursing. For example, some nurses who want the opportunity to practice massage in nursing receive training in massage schools and open private practices in order to provide the services they love. The rest of this book explores how nurses demonstrate caring, how complementary therapies have historically been an integral part of the science and art of nursing, and how some of these therapies can continue to be part of and support an integrative nursing practice in which the core values of caring, treating persons as individuals, and seeking wholeness in life, will be demonstrated through the caring modalities used in healing relationships with patients.

References

Brown, W. A. (1998). The placebo effect. *Scientific American* (January), 90–95.

Eisenberg, D. (1993). Unconventional medicine in the United States. *New England Journal of Medicine, 328* (4), 246–252.

Engebretson, J. (1996). Comparison of nurses and alternative healers. *IMAGE: Journal of Nursing Scholarship, 28* (2), 95–99.

Engel, G. L. (1977). The need for a new medical model: A challenge for biomedicine. *Science, 196,* 129.

Erlen, J. (1994). Technology's seductive power. *Orthopedic Nursing, 13* (6), 50–52.

Gordon, S. (1997). What nurses stand for. *The Atlantic Monthly,* (February), 80–88.

Hufford, D. (1997). Integrating complementary and alternative medicine into conventional medical practice. *Alternative Therapies, 3* (3), 81–83.

International Conference on Integrative Medicine (1999). <http://www.integrativemed.com>.

Macrae, J. (1995). Nightingale's spiritual philosophy and its significance for modern nursing. *IMAGE: Journal of Nursing Scholarship, 27* (1), 8–10.

May, C., & Fleming, C. (1997). The professional imagination: Narrative and the symbolic boundaries between medicine and nursing. *Journal of Advanced Nursing, 25,* 1094–1100.

Merriam-Webster's collegiate dictionary (10th ed.). (1999). Springfield, MA: Merriam-Webster.

Nightingale, F. (1969). *Notes on nursing.* New York: Dover.

Office of Alternative Medicine. (*What is CAM?* [Web Page]. URL http://altmed.od.nih.gov/oam [1998, August].

Peplau, H. (1988). The art and science of nursing: Similarities, differences and relations. *Nursing Science Quarterly, 1,* 8–15.

Pert, C. (1997). *Molecules of emotion: Why you feel the way you feel.* New York: Scribner.

Rinomhota, A. S., & Cooper, K. (1996). Homeostasis: Restoring the internal wellbeing in patients/clients. *British Journal of Nursing, 5* (18), 1100–1108.

Smith, M. (1994). Beyond the threshold: Nursing practice in the next millennium. *Nursing Science Quarterly, 7* (1), 6–7.

Sodestrom, K. E. & Martinson, I. M. (1987). Patient's spiritual coping strategies: A study of nurse and patient perspectives. *Oncology Nursing Forum, 14* (2), 41–45.

Tuck, I., Pullen, L., & Lynn, C. (1997). Spiritual interventions provided by mental health nurses. *Western Journal of Nursing Research, 19* (3), 351–363.

Watson, J. (1995). Nursing's caring-healing paradigm as exemplar for alternative medicine? *Alternative Therapies, 1* (3), 64–69.

DEMONSTRATING CARE

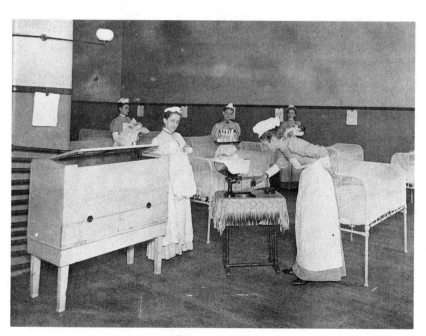

The nursery, 1895
(Courtesy Center for the Study of the History of Nursing, University of Pennsylvania.)

In Part One we discussed the major components of integrative nursing:

1. Weaving together biomedical skill and caring modalities in a practice that focuses on the creation of collaborative, healing relationships.
2. Assisting a patient to achieve and maintain balance or homeostasis.
3. Observing patients closely and providing holistic care for each individual patient.

These three components represent the theoretical foundation and overall picture of integrative nursing practice. At the heart of the integrative practice is the demonstration of caring to patients, which involves the modality, technique, or therapy used when caring for the patient (*what* we do) and the details of the way in which the care is demonstrated (*how* we do it).

Part Two focuses on the general concept of the *how* and *what* of demonstrating care. Chapter 3 discusses the caring event in greater detail, such as the nurse's source of strength for care, the effort involved in caring behavior, the influence of culture and health belief on demonstrating care, and complementary therapies in nursing practice.

Chapter 4 discusses the history of how nurses have demonstrated caring by highlighting ten nurses' narrative accounts regarding their own perceptions of how they, in their own nursing specialties, have demonstrated care. Chapter 5 discusses the potential future of caring.

As all three chapters address the *what* and *how* of demonstrating caring, it should become apparent why every nurse needs a "vehicle," if you will, for her caring spirit. Nurses need a modality or technique that harnesses their feelings toward another person and that enables them to communicate the understanding, compassion, empathy, and care they feel in their hearts. There are numerous modalities and treatments for which nurses have an affinity. Each caring modality can create a sense of hope, inspiration, power, and care in the caregiver as well as in the patient.

Many cultures, such as the Native American culture, believe that true "medicine" is in the healer, not in the modality used by the healer. While some nurses may find this to be true, patients do place value on the healing modalities used by nurses. Therefore, it is important to explore the caring modalities nurses use and their potential to be a powerful means of initiating healing relationships and conveying healing thoughts, feelings, and energy to a patient.

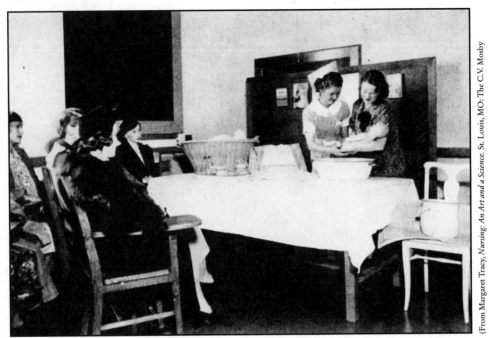

Parenting class, 1938

(From Margaret Tracy, *Nursing: An Art and a Science*. St. Louis, MO: The C.V. Mosby Company, 1938. Used with permission.)

Common sense is not so common.

—Voltaire

CHAPTER 3

Where Theories End and the Action Begins

Caring Moments

Caring is a process in which there is no definite beginning or ending. Caring implies a relationship between two people. Because caring and the caring relationship are always in process or in a state of becoming, they represent the ambiguity that the biomedical world works so diligently to control and eradicate. There is no predefined direction for the caring process. Despite the inherent ambiguity, nurses are often quite comfortable and even inspired by the caring process.

Trying to define the often ambiguous process of caring as what happens between two people reminded me of a time I experienced a similar struggle. I remember my sense of confusion about doing pirouettes, the turns in ballet. I was studying ballet with a teacher in New York City. I had spent years "trying" to turn. Although I could pirouette, it always felt forced and difficult. One day my teacher said to me, "A turn is what happens between two other movements. It's a moment in time between two movements and it just happens." After that, I stopped thinking about the turn as something I did. I just filled the music between two movements with turns, sometimes one, sometimes many more. The spirit of the dance directed how many turns happened and sometimes I was startled to find myself doing three times as many turns as the day before in the same given amount of time. In other words, the relationship of the turn to the rest of the dance changed for me.

What happens in healing relationships between a nurse and a patient is much like a pirouette. We can prepare for it, we can train to do it, but when it comes down to actually doing it and having it flow, we are not really in control of *it*. Caring occurs between two people the way a turn occurs between two movements. Caring is a manifestation of the spirit of our action as well as the action itself.

Sometimes theories about caring in nursing practice feel like a world of turns, somewhere between point A and point B. Many nurses ask how someone can learn caring by reading caring theory. They say that nurses either are, or are not, caring by nature. Again, the premise of this book is that all nurses are naturally caring people. The way a nurse is able to demonstrate, or put into practice, her caring spirit is what distinguishes each and every nurse. Each nurse's demonstration of caring is as unique as the individual. It is indeed possible to learn and become an expert in the demonstration of care to others. In fact, that is what nursing education is about.

Nursing action, the *what* and *how* of demonstrating care, is vitally important to integrative nursing practice. Although at times the theoretical underpinnings of *care* seem so shrouded in mystery, the actions of caring are not. It is to this part of the theory of human caring that I turn your attention.

Jean Watson, who developed one theory of human caring, writes, "The ideal and value of caring is clearly not just a *thing* out there, but is a starting point, a stance, an attitude, which has to become a will, an intention, a commitment, and a conscious judgement that manifests itself in concrete *acts*. . . . Human care can be effectively demonstrated and practiced only interpersonally" (Watson, 1988, pp. 31–33). It is these interpersonal acts that nurses perform with others that demonstrate their caring spirit. An act of genuine caring, regardless of its seeming simplicity, is important.

People are often so busy these days that it can take an act of caring and kindness, rather than just a kind word, to show that people care. For example, when I worked as a nurse and manager for a large pediatric practice we often had mothers come into the office with their children, carrying diaper bags, toys, snacks, etc. They were truly Herculean in that they could carry everything they did. The nursing staff decided to show these mothers we cared about them by making it our policy to help them carry their belongings from the waiting room to the office. In addition, we would give them frequent updates on the progress of the doctor if we were running late. We demonstrated that we appreciated the effort it took for these mothers to come in for appointments. It really helped diminish the amount of anxiety the mothers experienced during their visits.

Nurses have many such occasions to demonstrate caring. "Society needs the caring professions, and nursing in particular, to help to restore humanity and nourish the human soul in an age of technology, scientism, loneliness, rapid change and stresses, an age without moral or ethical wisdom, as to how to serve humanity (Watson, 1988, p. 49). Caring is often remembered as an event in the lives of those involved. The recipient rarely forgets genuine caring demonstrated from the heart. Watson says that "an actual caring occasion involves action and choice both by the nurse and by the individual. The moment of coming together in a caring occasion presents the two persons with the opportunity to decide how to be in the relationship—what to do with the moment. . . . The moment of the caring occasion becomes part of the past life history of both persons and presents both with new opportunities. What we all learn from it is self-knowledge. The self we learn about or discover is every self: it is universal—the human self. We learn to recognize ourselves in others" (Watson, 1988, p. 59).

This ability to recognize ourselves in others is the ability to empathize with our fellow human beings. Having feelings such as empathy and caring for another is what makes our caring actions genuine and believable. Integrative nursing practice embraces a philosophy of holistic care that demands commitment, will, empathy with the human condition, and genuine caring on the part of the nurse.

Effort and Overcare

How and when a nurse chooses to demonstrate caring is very personal. Because caring is about relationships, it is important that nurses understand the full impact and influence that they themselves and their *presence* in the healing relationship have on the healing experience of the patient. My personal experience has been that, when a healing relationship is established, I often receive healing as well as the patient. For example, I once experienced tremendous anguish over the loss of a relationship. During the time of grief, I was given a sense of hope every time I worked with patients and felt the simple human-to-human connection. I know that I received healing on many levels even though I was in a healing relationship in which I was the "healer." I ultimately realized through my work with patients that my anguish was really about loneliness rather than the loss of a specific friend. Nurses often identify themselves as the healer, the worker, and the giver in healing relationships. It is sometimes difficult to admit that it is part of the human condition to have our own needs for connection. Recognizing this helps put nurses in contact with feelings of empathy for others. Although each person in the healing relationship may have similar needs, the nurse and patient have different roles. The nurse takes on the role of health care provider and healer.

The healer in the relationship is an electrode for healing thoughts, energy, emotions, and strength. The healer can also be a cool, calm reflecting pool that the patient can use to get a clearer picture of what is going on in his life. These metaphors are reminders that we are active participants in the healing experience of the patients and that the energy and power of healing comes through the nurse as well as the patient. Even though we may not deliberately seek healing in the nurse-patient relationship, we can receive the benefits of the healing energy that enters our hearts. I have found that I am often energized and healed in the process of being a caregiver, witness, and participant in the healing of many patients.

Gunilla Astrom studied skilled nurses who were asked about their caring experiences. They too said that "it was worth caring because caring itself gave them satisfaction and pleasure. They saw it as a reward and a stimulation when they could help the patient and felt comfortable when their own caring discernment was of value for example in physician decisions" (Astrom, Norberg, & Hallberg, 1995, p. 114). Caring for another person can be an invigorating, stimulating, satisfying, and healing experience for a nurse. It also has the potential to be a draining and unhappy experience. What is it that makes the experience uplifting and healing? How does a nurse know when she has given too much? What are the "professional boundaries" in caregiving? Cultural and personal differences make it difficult to answer these questions for all nurses at all times. In general, though, there are two concepts that can help nurses create uplifting, healing relationships: overcare and effort.

OVERCARE

In nursing work there are endless opportunities to help others in need. Nursing is a service profession. Match up a group of caring, service-oriented professionals with a population with endless needs and it's only a matter of time until the energy is drained from the caregiver. For this reason, nurses must be able to set limits about when they can and cannot provide services to others. Nurses must be able to determine when their work is draining, instead of energizing, as well as understand what the process of caring is all about. Nurses who do not recognize that they have allowed themselves to be "drained" are like a car that runs out of gas; the drain is often due to overcare.

In *The Hiddden Power of the Heart,* Sara Paddison has defined "overcare" like this: "If care is oil for your system, then overcare is an oil leak. . . . Overcare will drain you physically, emotionally, mentally and spiritually. Overcare can be caused by right motives—real care taken to inefficient extremes. It can be caused by wrong motives, like worrying if someone is going to get a better job, car, or bonus than you. Ambition, competition and expectancy are all examples of overcare motivated by the head. Stress rules the planet and overcare is one of the field generals in disguise. The planet is starving for true, balanced care" (Paddison, 1995, pp. 222–223).

Nurses must care for others only inasmuch as the experience is balancing and energizing. If a nurse gets to the point where he is worried, extremely stressed, or feeling burned out and drained, a change must be made. Some shift has to occur. Imagine a healing relationship as a scale with two trays on either side of a pole. The caregiver and the care receiver are on opposite sides of the scale. If the nurse gives so much that the scale becomes unbalanced she experiences an energy shift or drain. A change must be made or the relationship may have to end because the caregiver can no longer give. Making a change does not necessarily mean that the nurse cannot take care of a patient, or that she has to quit her job! Stress is everywhere, and so is overcare. The answer to achieving balance is inside each caregiver. Each healing relationship requires time to learn how to maintain balanced care. With each patient, a nurse evaluates how much care is draining and how much is energizing. This is different for each relationship.

Many nurses have had the experience of a draining, overcaring relationship with a patient, family member, a community, or an organization. At one time I was an excessive overcarer. I not only overcared for my patients, but also overcared for the entire institution I worked for. I worried about administrative decisions that I had no control over and I even got stressed that I thought I had no control. Then I remembered that nurses are in control about who, where, and when they care for someone else. Nurses are in control of whether or not the caring experiences they enter into are energizing and inspiring. Nurses choose to observe their own actions and reactions and determine, each and every moment, where they are on the caring scale. Integrative nursing is about balance, harmony, and homeostasis, not just within the patient but within the caregiver as well.

Researchers such as Harvard psychologist David McClelland have shown, through increased salivary IgA production, that feelings of care enhance a person's immune system (McClelland & Kirshnit, 1988). Overcare experiences that cause excessive internal stress states have the ability to take us out of physical balance very quickly, making us unable to "feel good" about what we do or why we do it. In nursing, we can easily feel "double binded" in that we know we are supposed to *be* caring and *demonstrate* caring, yet we have not been taught how to care without overcaring. Many nurses shut off their caring feelings and stop pursuing caring experiences out of a natural, self-preservation mechanism, trying to maintain their own balance. Perhaps the goal should be to demonstrate caring in a balanced way so that this cycle of care-overcare-burnout is not created in the first place.

Knowing what the difference is between care and overcare is very personal to each individual nurse. It takes self-knowledge to understand our range of abilities as caregivers. One key to self-knowledge is to understand the *effort* behind our caring interactions with others. There is actually an entire science dedicated to the study of the effort or "how we concentrate our exertion" (Dell, 1977, p. 11). This science is called "movement analysis" or "movement description."

MOVEMENT ANALYSIS

Around the time of World War II, a movement scientist and analyst named Rudolf Laban developed the science of understanding and notating the qualitative changes that occur in movement and behavior (Laban & Lawrence, 1947). In my dance education I studied this system of analysis. Because nursing is a behavioral science, I have been applying this knowledge to my care of patients as well.

Upon entering the nursing profession, I realized, as did Laban when he applied his science to British industry, that each person, each caregiver, has her own movement profile or repertoire. Pause for a moment and think of the way you enter a patient's room when bringing something such as a medication or a meal tray. Some nurses gently knock on the door, quietly enter the room, and quickly set the object down. Other nurses knock quickly on the door, rush into the room, and stop at the bedside to slowly place the object down while commenting to the patient. We are all different in how we do things and we are all different in how we demonstrate caring to others. *No one way is better or worse than another.* We are all different just as our patients are all different. It is actually beneficial to patients that nurses are all so different because one might be better at demonstrating care to one patient as opposed to another. We connect differently with each patient. This can be observed through movement and understanding the efforts behind the actions.

Through studying movement profiles, including the effort contained in the movement, Laban found that certain combinations of individuals work better than others. This idea was used in British industry to create worker teams. Many people have had an experience working with someone with whom they "resonated." Things just flow when working with someone who complements your movement style. Movement style is linked to personality, and certain personalities are attracted to one another. Personalities often determine the nature of relationships. The patient and nurse's personalities and movement styles define the healing relationship.

Taking some of the guesswork out of what type of interaction is most effective for a particular patient can be helpful. Perhaps if a nurse had some understanding of her natural "efforts" related to her personality, she would be able to apply that understanding to her interactions with patients. This is just what Laban did with factory workers to create effective teams. As a nurse learns to recognize her effort or exertion patterns, it is possible for her to develop a repertoire of efforts that addresses the needs of many different types of patients, all with their own unique movement profiles and personalities. New efforts can be learned. "Movement quality is an aspect of behavior and can be considered a product of learning, metabolism, perception of the environment, whatever your particular bias is about what produces differences in behavior" (Dell, 1977, p. 12). Effort in movement is not necessarily a conscious process, but can become so with attention to how the actions occur. The following is a brief summary of the concept of effort so that you can begin to think about how you act with others, what your natural movement style is, and how you might expand your effort repertoire when demonstrating care to others.

There are four "ingredients" to assess when thinking of movement style, exertion, or effort: flow, weight, time, and space (Dell, 1977). The changes that occur in each factor occur in a range between two extremes. Effort is always assessed as to its appropriateness for a given situation and is not judged as right or wrong.

FLOW.   The extremes of flow are qualities of being "bound" or "free" and they represent the degree of *tension* in movement; bound flow being more tense and free being more relaxed. Neither free nor bound flow is "better" than the other. Dell gives the example of the bull in the china shop as an inappropriate use of free flow and of carefully carrying a pot of hot coffee as an example of appropriate use of restricted or bound flow.

WEIGHT.   The qualities of weight are strong and light, again representing two extremes. Dell says, "As you observe changes in the quality of weight in people around you, you may find that people sometimes deal with themselves, with one another or with many objects as if they were either large pieces of furniture or delicate paper flowers" (Dell, 1977, p. 21). My personal tendency is to be more delicate with people, especially with the infants who are often my patients. But delicate or light nonverbal movement expression is not "understood" by all patients, even babies. I am often called upon to express myself in a "strong" way. Another example of the shift from light to strong expression would be the nurse who gently touches a premature infant in an isolette and then has to provide CPR because the baby's heart stops. In this case the nurse's movement pattern not only becomes more "strong" but it also becomes more "quick."

TIME.   Time is observed as a range of movement between quickness and sustainment. These qualities are not used to measure rate of speed in movement but are more descriptive of the "qualitative changes toward" sustainment or quickness of movement. "The qualities of quickness and sustainment can occur and be observed when 'speed' is irrelevant and/or impossible to measure" (Dell, 1977, p. 26). An example of appropriate use of time would be when a nurse slows his walking pace to match the pace of an elderly patient he is escorting. Matching pace is one way to mirror a patient's nonverbal behavior. Mirroring is one way to enter the "world" of the patient. Patients who feel understood nonverbally often exhibit behaviors that nurses might interpret as "being more comfortable." A patient's comfort level is one way of telling if the appropriate effort qualities are in use by the caregiver.

SPACE.   The final factor, space, is sometimes indicated through visual contact or attention to that which is in one's space. "Movement in which spatial attention consists of overlapping shifts in the body among a number of foci, we call indirect. Movement in which spatial attention in the body is pinpointed, channeled, single focused we call direct. Indirect and direct are the elements or qualities of the space factor" (Dell, 1977, p. 29). Some patients choose to make eye contact with caregivers and some do not. Some patients' body movements, not just their eyes, demonstrate directness or indirectness.

When all four factors are put together in differing combinations and different intensities and levels of presentation, it can be seen that there are endless combinations and possibilities for developing a repertoire of movements to be used in the demonstration of caring behavior. This repertoire becomes especially important when, as nurses, we interact with patients from cultures other than our own. Movement patterns and nonverbal communication are very different from culture to culture. For example, a nurse may grow up in a culture in which touching a stranger is forbidden out of respect for the other person. She may communicate a tension flow of containment or bound flow when she is caring for patients. Then she is assigned care of a patient who is from a culture in which touch is reassuring and is considered a demonstration of care and respect. What does the nurse do? The importance of the nurse's ability to adapt her behavior and draw from a large *repertoire* of movement becomes quite clear if the goal of the nurse is to be able to demonstrate care in a "language" the patient understands.

Culture and Demonstrating Care

Dr. Madeline Leininger has written extensively on the subject of human caring, especially regarding transcultural nursing practice. If, in the practice of integrative nursing, one of the goals is to interact with patients in a holistic way, the nurse must not only be aware of the patient's movement patterns, but also his cultural beliefs and practices. The nurse's knowledge of the patient's culture supports the healing relationship. Dr. Leininger writes, "The third critical issue related to care is the diverse way that it is expressed by the actions of nurses and clients of different cultures in the world. There are marked cultural differences and some similarities in the ways nurses give care and in the way clients expect it to be given. The author's study of thirty cultures clearly indicates that differences are more prevalent than universals" (Leininger, 1988, p. 9).

It is impossible for a nurse to understand all the cultures she interacts with on a day-to-day basis, especially if we understand that culture does not just refer to race. When nurses refer to culturally sensitive nursing practice we are often speaking of race but *culture* is a much broader term. Different religious groups represent different "cultures." Age represents a different culture, as do different familial and socio-economic groups. Nurses can potentially interact with many different cultural groups on a daily basis (see Figure 3–1).

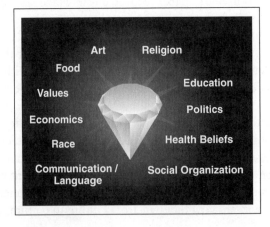

FIGURE 3-1
Facets of culture

I once worked at a children's hospital on an infant specialty care unit. The hospital was down the street from one church's headquarters and we often had babies on the unit who lived at the headquarters with their parents. The parents placed signs on the baby's cribs reminding staff not to discuss "negative thoughtforms" (i.e., anything regarding the illness of the baby) within hearing distance of the baby. This was an unusual request for me at the time, but very important to the families I was working with. From the experience, I learned a lot about this religious group. I actually found the practice of monitoring what I say near babies to be appropriate caring practice for my work with all babies. My way of demonstrating care changed after this experience. I actually became quite sensitive to the way nurses talk to and around babies. I have experienced nurse colleagues who are also careful about their comments to their infant patients, as well as to other colleagues and family members when in the presence of a baby.

Being observant of cultural differences and similarities enables us to expand our awareness of ourselves as nurses and as human beings. The process of addressing cultural caring needs is just another way of demonstrating care. It may be a subtle change, such as how I changed what I discussed near my infant patient, or it may be a much larger change.

Being willing to change behavior and movement style is key to integrative nursing practice that respects and supports the individual needs of patients. "Focusing on the patient and respecting the patient's lifeplan are ways the nurse demonstrates caring. Caring means that something is important and that something matters" (Erlen, 1994, p. 52). Caring activities are personalized to the needs of the individual patient receiving the care as well as the individual nurse providing the care. Demonstrating care as a process and a range of possibility is very personal. It is a process that takes introspection and understanding of one's own personality, movement style, ability to change and grow, and understanding of the process of balanced, energizing caregiving. This process also includes understanding the health beliefs that we bring to all healing relationships.

Complementary Therapies and Health Beliefs

As nurses explore the cultural needs and health beliefs of patients, they discover the numerous ways people heal themselves. The list of complementary therapies in Appendix A includes many modalities and practices that have been part of the health beliefs and health practices of different cultures for many years. Included are acupuncture from China and ayurveda from India. There are numerous therapies such as massage, other forms of touch therapies, faith healing, and herbal medicines, that are found in the health practices of many cultures though they may differ slightly in how they are used in nursing practice.

Because of the link between complementary therapies and different cultures' healing traditions, it is important that nurses who wish to practice integrative nursing not dismiss these healing practices now being spoken of as complementary or alternative.

The term itself implies the domination of the biomedical "culture." It also implies that all healing practices that are not part of the biomedical "culture" are alternative or complementary. It is true that the Eisenberg study found that 83 percent of the Americans surveyed had seen a doctor as well as an alternative therapist for a particular condition (1993). But who can say that in the patient's mind the biomedical therapy was the primary or most valued therapy. What if the biomedical treatment is secondary to the CAM therapy in the patient's view? How does a nurse know and why should she care?

If nurses are to demonstrate care effectively, in the "language" of the patient, they must identify the needs of the individual patient. It is often difficult for patients entering the biomedical culture's establishments (a hospital, public health office, or nursing home) to verbalize a need for care that has been labeled "alternative and complementary." This is no different from a nurse sitting in a room filled with physicians discussing a patient from a medical perspective and the nurse feeling somewhat intimidated by the thought of trying to broach the subject of care when everyone else is having an excited discussion over the newest cure. It wouldn't be surprising if the nurse just sat and listened. I have seen the same thing with patients who use a complementary therapy and would like to discuss with their caregivers how the therapy or modality has helped them. But the common feeling among many patients who use complementary therapies is that their doctors and nurses are not interested in what they are doing and "do not believe" in that sort of thing.

Although there have been some studies on this topic, I have experienced this firsthand as a practitioner for fifteen years of what is now called alternative and complementary therapies. The people who came to me for help all told me the same story. They do not tell their primary care provider about what they are doing because they do not want to alienate their provider. They often told me that their doctor and nurse "look down" on the other therapies they use in healing.

Many nurses and physicians are not aware of their cultural biases toward biomedicine. Biomedicine is one of many health belief systems and it is important that nurses understand that the public often views nurses as part of the biomedical culture, not as a separate nursing culture. If our goal is to provide integrative care for the public, then we need to understand their health decisions and the beliefs upon which they base their health decisions. We must understand and respect that people who value caring modalities and CAM therapies as first-line healing practices base their health decisions upon sound reasoning, just as those who value conventional biomedicine as a first-line healing practice do, and are deserving of our respect.

Dr. Bonnie O'Connor, an ethnographer who has studied various cultures' health beliefs, and how health decisions are made, writes that people who participate in healing practices other than the conventional practices of biomedicine use the same reasoning process when making their health decisions as those who use biomedicine.

People of highly diverse persuasions and backgrounds seem to reason to their conclusions in much the same fashion—building stepwise upon their axiomatic foundations and subsequent learning, taking into account their evidence, including observation and personal experience, and testing possibilities and hypotheses: making inferences, and accepting, rejecting and modifying various propositions as they go. The different conclusions reached within various belief systems do not appear to stem from incapacity to reason, nor from fundamentally different uses of reason. They may simply result from different observations, or differing interpretations of the same observation. (p. 13)

Conclusion

Listening to patients and encouraging them to express their thoughts, concerns, and beliefs about their health is a way of demonstrating caring and a way of developing healing relationships with patients. Nurses who value the individuality of patients and respect their health care choices are better able to provide integrative care.

Much has been written and discussed about caring. What caring *is* and can *become* is truly personal to each nurse-patient relationship. Caring happens in the *effort* that accompanies the nursing intervention. Caring can be part of any nursing activity, regardless of the choice of treatment, modality, therapy, or intervention. The sky's the limit!

References

Astrom, G., Norberg, A., & Hallberg, I. (1995). Skilled nurses' experience of caring. *Journal of Professional Nursing, 11* (2), 110–118.

Dell, C. (1977). A primer for movement description (2nd ed.). New York: Dance Notation Bureau.

Eisenberg, D. (1993). Unconventional medicine in the United States. *New England Journal of Medicine, 328* (4), 246–252.

Erlen, J. (1994). Technology's seductive power. *Orthopedic Nursing, 13* (6), 50–52.

Laban, R. & Lawrence, F. C. (1947). *Effort.* London: McDonald and Evans (out of print).

Leininger, M. (1988). *Care: The essence of nursing and health.* Detroit, MI: Wayne State University Press.

McClelland, D. & Kirshnit, C. (1988). The effect of motivational arousal through films on salivary immunoglobulin. *Psychology and Health, 2,* 31–52.

O'Connor, B. B. (1995). *Healing traditions: Alternative medicine and the health professions.* Philadelphia: University of Pennsylvania Press.

Paddison, S. (1995). *The hidden power of the heart: Achieving balance and fulfillment in a stressful world.* Boulder Creek, CA: Planetary Publications.

Watson, J. (1988). *Nursing: Human science and human care.* New York: National League for Nursing.

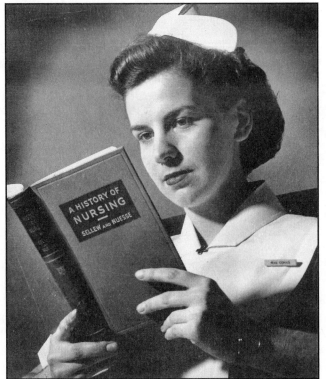

Looking through the history book

I solemnly pledge myself before God and in the presence of this assembly, to pass my life in purity and to practice my profession faithfully. I will abstain from whatever is deleterious and mischievous, and will not take or knowingly administer any harmful drug. I will do all in my power to maintain and elevate the standard of my profession, and will hold in confidence all personal matters committed to my keeping and all family affairs coming to my knowledge in the practice of my calling. With loyalty will I endeavor to aid the physician in his work, and devote myself to the welfare of those committed to my care.

—MRS. LYSTRA E. GRETTER, RN,
"THE FLORENCE NIGHTINGALE PLEDGE" (1893)

CHAPTER 4

How Nurses Demonstrate Caring: Past and Present

Nursing theorists such as Jean Watson and Madeline Leininger have addressed the importance of caring to nursing in their writings. They have elaborately described the philosophical and theoretical underpinnings of caring as a foundation for nursing practice. Understanding caring in this way is important to deepen the understanding of the goals and mission of the profession.

Caring Modalities

It is also important for nurses to understand the practical application of caring theory and philosophy. In order to apply caring theory to practice, a nurse must choose caring modalities or actions, often equated with comfort measures, that she finds effective. The nurse must also choose caring acts, or modalities, that the patient will perceive as caring. It is this *choice* of the caring modality that provides the nurse with the opportunity for creativity and self-expression as a healer.

Having received my nursing education from Mount St. Mary's College in the early 1980s, I was educated in the "nursing process." I learned that before intervening and providing care for a patient, I must first assess the patient's needs and then formulate a plan of care. I learned that the job of the nurse is then to work with the patient to decide how the patient's needs will be met. These caring measures, treatments, or acts are what I will refer to as modalities.

The word *modality* is found in medical dictionaries. In Taber's Cyclopedic Medical Dictionary (1997), modality is defined as, "A method of application or the employment of any therapeutic agent. . . . Any specific sensory stimulus such as taste, touch, vision, pressure, or hearing." Throughout this chapter I will refer to nurses' caring actions, skills, and treatments used in caring for patients as modalities.

Nursing modalities are the "instruments" nurses use in their work with patients. Just as the physician in the biomedical world has technology and drugs as her instruments of healing, the nurse has caring modalities. These caring modalities are like a crystal chalice into which a precious elixir of caring feelings, thoughts, and efforts are poured. The effectiveness of the caring modality is determined by its ability to harness the energy of the love and compassion stored in the heart of the nurse and the patient, which can then be used for healing.

There are a wealth of caring modalities that have been used in nursing practice throughout history. Many of these modalities are a product of different cultures and different understandings of the healing process of the body. It is important to look at nursing history and caring modalities as we begin the new millennium and as we make personal and professional decisions about what nursing is and what it is not.

History of Caring Modalities

As is stated in the nurses' pledge of 1893 at the beginning of this chapter, nurses have spent many years as the assistant and supporter to biomedical practitioners. Although this may continue to be the case to some degree, it is important for nurses to continue to strive for greater definition of the unique way in which caring modalities are used in nursing practice. This chapter explores the history of caring modalities and their presence in nursing practice today. As we look to the future of nursing and begin to formulate a vision of what nursing practice will look like, it is important to understand the past and its impact on the present. The study of the past often provides a sense of reassurance and continuity. In today's health care environment, reassurance and continuity are often sorely needed.

People and cultures observe their histories and past discoveries in different ways. This is true about the history of health care discovery as well. For instance, when I studied Chinese herbal medicine, I learned that the Chinese never toss aside any of their theories of healing just because they come up with a new theory. I learned a theory of assessment called eight principle patterns, which is a theory that is thousands of years old. This theory teaches the understanding of the overall qualities of a patient related to heat, cold, interior, exterior, excess, deficiency, yin, and yang. It is interesting that many of the modalities used historically in nursing are based on theories of heat, cold, deficiency, and excess as well. When the Chinese created new theories, such as the five element theory so often used today in American schools of acupuncture, they did not stop using older theories, such as the eight principle patterns, but considered all theories to be relevant to the growing knowledge base of health care science.

During the expansion of the biomedical era in the West, as well as today, health beliefs held by physicians and nurses not that long ago are often considered ancient, outdated, and irrelevant. Affluent developed nations can usually afford to discard the older health beliefs and practices that were often simple and inexpensive by today's standards. Nations such as China could not. China made a decision years ago that, due to economic and other reasons, they could not rely solely upon the new medicine from the West.

Western biomedicine has been exported to the East for decades. But China is not alone in its inability to finance a complete shift away from historical health care practices. Biomedicine is expensive for many nations. As C. Everett Koop, former Surgeon General for the United States has said, "For years we have attempted to export Western medicine to the developing world. The sad truth is that the people we are attempting to help simply cannot afford it. I have doubts about how much longer we can afford some of it ourselves. It is possible that a decade from now, we may be more ready to ask the peoples of the developing world to share their wisdom with us" (Micozzi, 1996, pp. x–xi). Perhaps this wisdom sharing between East and West is part of the emergence of integrative practice. Many nations have strong traditional healing practices that exist side by side with biomedical practice. It is helpful to have at least an understanding of the traditional healing practices of a culture, and how they may be integrated with aspects of biomedicine, when trying to establish healing relationships.

How nurses integrate biomedical and caring modalities is demonstrated in the way they care for patients. Nurses seldom record the work that has been done in this regard. Although nursing history often records the individual accomplishments and contributions of nursing leaders, little has been written on how nurses have demonstrated caring throughout history, the modalities that have been used in the care of patients, and how these may or may not have changed throughout the years. "A search throughout ancient history reveals little, however, about attendants to the sick—nurses. This may be because unusual or striking events rather than ordinary ones are generally recorded in history. People have always nursed their sick as a matter of course. It was not until cities became large and problems became acute that the matter of care in illness warranted specific mention. Yet one can be reasonably sure that nurses, male or female, functioned in early civilization. . . . The history of India reveals a more complete description of nursing principles and practice than that of any other civilization. Throughout the historical documents of India frequent references are made to nurses. In most instances these nurses were men; however in rare cases they were old women" (Donahue, 1996, pp. 30, 48).

Although we know some things about nursing history, such as that much of the nursing care in Europe was historically provided by the religious orders, little information is provided in historical texts as to the modalities used by nurses until the publication of nursing textbooks of the late 1800s or early 1900s. "Little is known about the actual care given the sick during the Dark Ages. Secular medicine was almost completely extinguished, and there was little impetus toward advancement in the science and art of nursing or of medicine. In fact, little distinction was made between medicine and nursing" (Donahue, 1996, p. 102). It is from these nursing textbooks, called *materia medica* in some cases, from the 1800s and 1900s that a written explanation of the modalities used in nursing care can be found. As nursing care differentiates itself from medicine more and more, the need for an examination of nurses' caring modalities becomes more important.

Nursing Fundamentals in the Nineteenth and Twentieth Centuries

> It is accepted in informed circles that a critical evaluation of existing problems and sound solutions for them, current and in terms of future planning, are hardly possible without an understanding of related antecedents and a sufficient knowledge of historical development in its cause and effect relationships. This is particularly true of the problems of the nursing profession—a profession that not only has a science and art of its own but borrows from and coordinates the functions of several allied disciplines, all aimed at one great goal but dependent on nursing to a greater or lesser degree to make their functions effective for the people they serve. (Frank, 1959, p. 4)

The antecedents of present-day nursing practice can be found in the writings on nursing fundamentals in textbooks such as *Text-book of the Principles and Practice of Nursing* (1924) by Bertha Harmer, *Text-book of the Principles and Practice of Nursing* (1939) by Harmer and Virginia Henderson, *Nursing: An Art and a Science* (1938) by Margaret Tracy, and *Notes on Nursing,* originally written by Florence Nightingale in 1859. These historical texts depict the common foci in nursing practice, as well as the caring modalities used, from the late 1800s to the 1900s.

Florence Nightingale wrote a book about what might now be called the fundamentals of nursing practice or bedside care (Nightingale, 1969). She wrote about the importance of the well-ventilated room, diet, light, bedding, cleanliness, and observation of the sick. Margaret Tracy wrote about the fundamentals of nursing as being the nurse's "daily care," which included the bath, making the bed, care of the patient's mouth and hair, assistance with meals, preparation for sleep, and care of body wastes (Tracy, 1938, p. 73). She also said that, "Many additional services which the nurse renders to the patient are not matters of doctor's orders or of routine, but thoughtful contributions to his comfort and well-being which the observant nurse will make. In order to carry out the things which contribute to the comfort of the patient, the nurse first of all must have an understanding of people and their problems. The nurse should feel that it is an essential part of her care of the patient for her to know something about his history and background as a human being as well as the history of disease. Armed with this knowledge, she can give the patient a more sympathetic understanding which in turn will bring to him a sense of security and ease of mind" (p. 73). This encouragement of the "easing of the patient's mind" also spoken of by Tracy can be summed up in the Nightingale philosophy that encourages nurses to place the patient in the best possible condition for nature to work upon him." "Nature alone cures. Surgery removes the bullet out of the limb, but nature heals the wound. Medicine as far as we know, assists nature to remove the obstruction, but does nothing more. And what nursing has to do in either case, is to put the patient in the best condition for nature to act upon him. Generally, just the contrary is done. You think fresh air, and quiet and cleanliness extravagant, perhaps dangerous luxuries, which should be given to the patient only when quite convenient, and medicine the sine qua non, the panacea" (Nightingale, 1957, p. 75). Many of the historical nursing texts exemplify this work with nature by using water, by using plants as topical and internal medicines, and by adjusting the temperature, ventilation, and brightness of a room. This work with the patient's environment, as well as attending to their basic daily needs, has been called nursing fundamentals. Florence Nightingale seemed to define nursing fundamentals as those acts that supported the patient's relationship with nature, the provider of the cure.

Comfort Measures

Historical nursing texts also discuss the importance of demonstrating care by addressing the patient's comfort. Tracy says, "In thinking of her patient as a 'person' largely dependent on the nurse for his comfort, the nurse will then consider all of the things she can do to bring the most comfort to the patient" (p. 73). Each patient's comfort needs are unique. It takes skill in understanding others, as well as a repertoire of caring modalities, to address the unique needs of the individual patient. "The nurse should learn to think of every patient as an individual whose comfort lies in her hands. She should attempt to ascertain and, if possible, to remove causes of worry, confusion, strangeness, and discomfort which are hindering the progress of her patient" (Tracy, 1938, p. 93). Since the early years of nursing practice, it was understood that stressful emotions, such as worry and concern, compromised the healing ability of the patient. For this reason, the nurse was responsible for helping the patient find comfort, which is not as easy as it might seem. If one thinks only about the cultural variations in what is considered comforting, it is clearly a monumental task to provide the appropriate comfort for a given patient.

Many caring modalities have been created out of a need to find ways to comfort patients. Providing comfort can mean relieving pain, setting the mind at ease, and providing familiarity for the patient. This nursing task of providing comfort is critical to the health of the patient, especially when the patient is hospitalized or being cared for in an unfamiliar environment.

Even as, historically, nurses have recognized the importance of comfort, today we have the scientific understanding of the stress response to support the historical emphasis on comfort of patients. The stress response, also called fight or flight response, is the body's homeostatic response to a perceived life threat. This response primarily involves the sympathetic nervous system and the endocrine system. Adrenaline is released into the bloodstream causing pupil dilation, muscle tension, increased heart rate, peripheral vasoconstriction, and an elevation of blood pressure.

The liver also releases stored sugar, or glycogen, digestion is inhibited, and blood is diverted to the brain and muscles to prepare the body for attack. Unfortunately, the human body is not able to tolerate prolonged periods of fight or flight. What begins as a normal stress response becomes a threat to health, and potentially life itself, when experienced for long periods of time. For example, many people develop ulcers with prolonged periods of stress because the fight or flight response decreases the amount of protective mucus secreted by the stomach. With knowledge of the biological workings of the stress response, especially over long periods of time, the importance of keeping the normal response from being overstimulated cannot be overestimated, hence the importance of comfort, familiarity, and modalities that can aid a patient in maintaining a calm state rather than activating the fight or flight response, especially when they are ill already.

Nurses are aware of the numerous stressors patients experience when they have a challenging health situation. Many events occur during an illness that can activate the stress response: the diagnosis itself, a change in lifestyle, and a change in environment, to name a few. "There is no other field in the care of the sick in which the comfort and recovery of the patient are so dependent upon good nursing and no other field which so challenges or puts a nurse more upon her mettle or which offers such scope for mastering the difficult art and science of nursing. A good nurse is always at her best in taking care of patients suffering from such diseases . . . which by no means known to the art of man can abort or shorten, but in which nursing care can do much to alleviate, to prevent complications or to shorten convalescence. Such diseases are called the 'nurses patients,' the doctor being at hand only for general supervision" (Harmer, 1924, p. 325). Indeed many domains in health care have been influenced by nursing care. Many more areas could be better addressed by nurses.

Historical Narratives:
How Nurses Demonstrate Caring

In order to discover more about the modalities nurses use in demonstrating care and providing comfort to patients, I interviewed ten nurses who have been in practice for at least ten years. Five nurses were retired from nursing practice and five nurses were in practice. The nurses were asked ten questions about their nursing practice, how they have demonstrated caring to their patients over the years, and whether they have used the caring modalities outlined in historical texts on nursing fundamentals.

I wanted to explore the nurses' understanding of caring modalities, what they have found to "work" well with patients, and what they have done in practice that they have perceived as having been received as caring by their patients. My reasoning for choosing nurses who are retired or have been in practice for more than ten years is based upon a study by Astrom, Norberg, and Hallberg (1995). This study supported the importance of listening to skilled nurses' stories of caring. "This work describes practical implication, the usefulness of listening to skilled people's experiences. The nurses in this study revealed without hesitation their experiences of caring and were convinced that their experiences were important. It seems, therefore, essential to make room in the everyday practice for skilled nurses to narrate their experiences about caring for less experienced carers" (Astrom, Norberg, and Hallberg, 1995, p. 117). The content of the interviews was evaluated for any common themes about demonstrating care, both within the individual nurse's interviews as well as among all ten interviews.

I discovered that the modalities viewed as useful for demonstrating care were similar among the nurses interviewed. The nurses identified caring modalities they use today that are, in general, similar to the caring modalities discussed in historical nursing texts. It is my hope in sharing the narratives that you might identify those historical similarities as well as identify the many ways *you* demonstrate caring to patients. As discussed previously, there has been so little written on actual nursing practice because much of what we have done for years in taking care of people has seemed mundane, but, as we move forward and develop as a profession, it is important to listen to and study what nurses have found to be successful in administering care. In a technologically advanced world, we can develop and expand our knowledge of these established ways of demonstrating care much like the Chinese have done with some of their ancient healing modalities.

It is interesting that the findings of the Astrom study confirm the benefit of experienced nurses telling their stories to others. I have always benefited from learning from the experiences of my "elders." My hope is that whether you are an experienced or novice caregiver, you will benefit from hearing a little bit about these nurses' choices and caring actions. I also hope that your reflection on the stories of these nurses will encourage you to begin the process of reflection on your own abilities to demonstrate caring to patients, regardless of how long you have been a professional nurse.

How Ten Expert Nurses Demonstrate Care

The following section is a short synopsis of each of the narratives of the experienced nurses. Following the synopses is a brief analysis of the themes that emerged from the interviews and their potential relevance to nursing practice today. To keep the identities of these nurses confidential, I have used pseudonyms. The names I have given them are the names of saints from Western cultures. In my culture, it is an honor to name someone after a saint. According to the 1956 version of *Webster's New Collegiate Dictionary*, a saint is not only defined as one officially canonized, but can also be defined as someone who is "extraordinarily charitable, patient and self-denying. A saint is a holy or godly person" (*Webster's New Collegiate Dictionary,* 1956). Having heard these nurses and their career stories, I can witness to the fact that they are indeed "saints" in their own right.

BARBARA: SPECIALTY, ONCOLOGY.   Barbara found her "niche" in oncology nursing many years ago. She works in the high-tech world of powerful drugs. She works in a nursing world that "deals with the whole person, including the dying person." Barbara has experienced the feeling called "burnout" and says that, "In order to continue doing what I'm doing I have to put balance in my practice, so that I can give and I can also receive by giving. There's more of a reciprocal thing where I don't end up empty."

In sharing how she demonstrates caring, Barbara recognizes that starting IVs and other similar tasks are the "easy stuff" and that "what makes a difference is the human connection . . . being gentle, having a calming demeanor, and helping the patient's experience be as pain-free as possible." Barbara describes nursing as a "magic" that many, especially those in medicine, do not understand. This nursing magic includes the "powerful" act of being "present with a patient and the family . . . connecting with someone to the point where the rest of the world goes away for a moment." She says that her ability to be "present in the moment with a patient" is more important than any drug she gives. Being present is not easy for Barbara because the environments in which she works are very "distracting, rude, intrusive, cold, and sterile." She demonstrates caring by creating a "receiving environment" for the patient. She wants to create environments that are full of "life," but is often limited by the biomedical therapy the patient is undergoing. For example, people on chemotherapy cannot have live plants in their environment.

Barbara also talks about the importance of touch in her work with oncology patients. She demonstrates caring with hugs, especially after chemotherapy. She also uses warmed lotion to give back massages to patients whose "muscles are tired from lying in bed all day."

Barbara says that understanding a person's culture is important when providing care. For instance, she often discusses the patient's diet with him. She has learned to be creative in applying her "book" of knowledge about diet and chemotherapy and tailoring her suggestions to the individual patient. For example, she says, "The book says, 'no chiles when you're on chemotherapy,' but what about the Hispanic patient?" Other caring modalities Barbara uses are aromatherapy, color therapy, hydrotherapy, and relaxation therapy.

The most important moment in Barbara's career as a nurse was when, as a nurse's aide, she witnessed a death for the first time. She said, "I could feel the energy in the room change when she, the patient, died in my presence. It was very peaceful and I wasn't afraid of death from that moment on. Until that moment, I wasn't sure I could be a nurse. After that experience I knew that I could be okay with this whole profession. Nursing is more than a job; it's a lifestyle, a commitment. It's where I've put a lot of time and energy and a lot of myself into it. It's so hard to figure out how to integrate that into what's going on in any culture of nursing. I don't want to be tired when I work now. I want to be alert; I want to be attentive. I want to eat right and sleep right so that I can be a better nurse when I am a nurse."

FRANCES: SPECIALTY, MENTAL HEALTH/NURSING EDUCATION. Frances describes demonstrating care in nursing as "relationship building" and "establishing rapport" through therapeutic communication. Frances began her nursing career during wartime and says that she was responsible for hundreds of patients. She demonstrated caring by learning and remembering all of her patients' names. This really impressed patients and staff! She learned that listening to patients was very important and that, "Every interaction with a patient is an opportunity to listen to the patient and spend time with a patient." Frances recognizes that today's nurses work in organizations that place many demands on them. "I can tell you that over the years, this is not new. . . . We don't have much time, but nurses sometimes use the 'system' as an excuse for not caring."

When I asked Frances how she learned to communicate with patients she said that it was by observation of the nurses she worked with during her training as a nurse. She learned how to be "diplomatic" in her interactions with others. Frances also used the environment in her care of patients. She used tub baths to calm agitated patients and wrapped them in cold sheets. (The body's reaction to cold sheets is to quickly warm the exterior of the body, which can be very relaxing.) The nurses were also very careful about noises in the patients' environment as the soldiers often startled easily. Frances was also an expert in assisting with electric shock therapy. She has continued her interest in the use of energy in nursing care by learning therapeutic touch. She has been a therapeutic touch practitioner since 1978 and uses this modality in her nursing work. She has also used massage and effleurage.

AGATHA: SPECIALTY, POST-ANESTHESIA CARE UNIT (PACU). Agatha worked for the same organization for over thirty years. She believes that demonstrating care in nursing can be as simple as "putting a cool cloth on someone's forehead, spoonfeeding them water when they are having a hard time keeping anything down, and cradling them when they cry." Agatha calls these "nursing traits." She has also used touch to demonstrate care to patients.

Agatha recalls the importance of back rubs, foot soaks, shampooing heads, and holding a patient's hand. Because her patients were on heart monitors, she could see the slowing of the patient's heart rate when she offered caring touch. She also found that turning and positioning patients or walking with patients were some of the most important caring measures. Agatha describes demonstrating care through positioning patients as being more than "turning a patient from side to side . . . we used all the positions."

Agatha also believes that a nurse demonstrates caring by providing and assisting with the patient's meal. She says, "If a person isn't nourished, they don't heal." The nurse can demonstrate caring by making the food accessible, the right temperature, and attractive. She says that many patients are given food that is "overwhelming," such as a large "slab" of meat. Agatha always assisted her patients to receive "nourishment."

Agatha also describes demonstrating care as "honoring the patient." She encouraged the patient's "free expression" and really listened to the needs of patients and their families. If a family needed to pray together she gave them the privacy they needed. She also took opportunities to "be with a patient and listen to their stories." She took advantage of any time spent with a patient, even when giving them a bedpan, to get to know them a little more.

Agatha says that she has used massage, relaxation therapy, footbaths, and hand pressure points with her PACU patients over the years. She learned the healing power of the sun when she moved to Colorado years ago and saw people with tuberculosis being treated by solar therapy. She also believes that it is caring to provide nursing services that are patient-centered. Pain management is a big concern of nurses working in the PACU. Nurses often demonstrate care for the patient by providing timely and appropriate medication. Agatha said that before retiring she began to observe that patients seemed to have a greater need for narcotics. PACU patients sometimes do not remember that they have been given something for pain. She believes that nurses need to become more creative in finding ways to help patients deal with pain. "We rely on drugs to put the patient down and make them comfortable and I see that in the expectation of the patient also. The healing arts has fallen away to make room for all the science of nursing. . . . We can't compromise anymore."

JOAN: SPECIALTY, PEDIATRICS AND WOMEN'S PSYCHIATRY.   When Joan was asked how she demonstrates caring in her nursing practice, she recalled providing "TLC" to babies by patting, holding, and bathing them. She believes that "nurses must have hands-on experience" to be caregivers. She also found that talking with patients is important. One time she cried with parents whose child had just died. Although she was criticized by a nurse superior for behavior unbecoming a professional nurse, Joan believes to this day that at times it is appropriate to cry with families.

Joan also remembers demonstrating care for patients through touch. She learned how to give full body massages in nursing school. She also learned the Sister Kenny methods of treating polio, a hydrotherapy method using flannel and rubber sheets to wrap the body. Solariums were also used for polio patients. Joan was also taught how to use continuous baths to help calm a person. She also learned to use mustard plasters on the chest for colds and pneumonia.

Joan demonstrates caring by meeting patients "where they are." For example, she once took students into a nursing home for a clinical experience. There was a German woman in the nursing home who never spoke until one day when Joan made a special tape of old German folk songs and played it for the woman. The woman began singing with the tape and then spoke for the first time because the music was able to reach her. Joan's bright and compassionate ideas were well received by her patients. She believes that nurses are more than "workhorses, they are intelligent."

MARGARET: SPECIALTY, TRAVELING NURSE, MILITARY NURSE, RED CROSS.

Margaret "built her own career." She worked during the war and traveled with the navy by ship and train. She also taught for the Red Cross. Communication with patients, listening to them, and supporting them was how Margaret has demonstrated caring in her nursing practice. She remembers "long backrubs with patients . . . that was the only time they could really share. . . . I remember sitting on the bed talking to a patient and his wife. These things were kind of automatic and you just didn't think about the therapeutic value." In addition to back rubs, Margaret also knew the importance of a well-timed pat on the shoulder or a hug. She believes that it is the nurse who needs to provide opportunities for sharing.

Nutrition was also an important modality for Margaret. She taught classes to mothers about caring for babies and children in which nutrition was a big part of the curriculum. Margaret provided nursing care during a time when nurses provided flaxseed or mustard poultices to patients. Poultices are a topical application of a slurry of herbs with a cotton, linen, or wool cloth to a particular part of the body.

Margaret describes herself as a nurse who is "not assertive or noisy but who speaks her mind." She believes that "nursing and medicine are complementary and that they need to work together for the good of the patient."

ANNE: SPECIALTY, OBSTETRICS, SUBSTANCE MISUSE.

Anne describes her way of demonstrating care as a way of being with a patient. She says that she helps people make decisions and maintain control. For instance, she cites the example of taking a baby's temperature while resting in the mother's arms rather than having to take the baby from the mother. She also believes that caring is demonstrated by consulting patients and not making decisions for patients. She is nonjudgmental and does not like to "label" patients. She says, for example, that "We give the patient a *DSM-IV* diagnosis or label and then we often forget to look at the human suffering that they're going through."

Communication with patients has been very important to Anne. She connects with patients by active listening and creating an environment in which the patient feels comfortable to share her story. She provides a caring environment by making herself available to hear the woman's story of her labor experience. She says that, "The nurse creates an environment that a person can feel safe and comfortable in so that they can feel that they can be honest and express what it is they need to express . . . what they are really feeling." She demonstrates caring by "being" with a patient.

Anne has also used various modalities to demonstrate caring. She was part of a mental health team that used light therapy in the treatment of depressed patients. She has used hydrotherapy such as sitz baths, showers, and water birth, as well as massage and effleurage in her care of female patients. Anne has demonstrated caring to patients with relaxation techniques such as meditation. She has also found the 12-step program to be helpful in her care for patients.

MARY: SPECIALTY, MEDICAL SURGICAL/EDUCATION. When asked how she has demonstrated caring for patients over the years, Mary talked about her experience as a med-surg nurse during the war. She said that, "I had fifteen patients, no coffee breaks, and washed my hands in Lysol between each patient. We did not have time at that point to do much with the patient as a human being. World War II made a difference. After that patients were, and still are, treated like little soldiers." She talked about watching nursing care go to a "more chemical approach."

Back rubs, Mary said, were "one of the best things we ever did." A masseur taught her how to give a "real" back rub in nursing school. Different topical applications were used depending on the climate the patient was in. For example, alcohol and powder were used for back rubs in the eastern United States. The back rub was the best time to communicate with the patient. Mary believes that she demonstrated caring when she provided an opportunity for the patient to talk. A "nurse is a listener." She found that her relationships with patients were often very intimate.

She also demonstrated care with hydrotherapy such as hot packs, hot water bottles, and sponging and cooling (especially before there were antibiotics). She taught patients the importance of a well-balanced diet. She also remembers doctors ordering "spiritus fermentae" for patients—she gave them a glass of wine. Mary believes that she demonstrated caring by encouraging patients to "listen to their bodies." When asked if Mary learned this in school she said, "Oh no, we were taught to tell patients to listen to their doctors and we were to reinforce whatever the doctor said!"

CATHARINE: SPECIALTY, COMMUNITY HEALTH/PHONE NURSING. Catharine believes that she began to learn ways to demonstrate caring long before she even had formal nurses' training. She describes giving a person a urinal, giving a bed-bath, or providing a cup of coffee as "caring things." "Providing the little things needed for comfort are sometimes easier without a lot of education." Catharine's philosophy of nursing is that it is a combination of the "nurse as a person and their own caring aspects and their education." She believes that sometimes education is "intuitive rather than formal."

Touch is very important to Catharine's way of demonstrating care to patients. She talked about giving hugs when appropriate. She has held patients' hands both literally and now figuratively in her work as a phone nurse. Catharine is studying traditional Chinese medicine and has learned a lot about the importance of touch from her master teacher. She says that when the teacher touches her to demonstrate a pulse diagnosis, she can "feel his qi [Chinese word for the life force or energy in the body]. You can feel his caring when he touches you." Catharine demonstrates caring by being aware of the energy she conveys to others. She describes how as a young nurse she tried to make patients' needs conform to her schedule, such as making people wait to receive a pain medication until she got to their room when she was passing out medications. She says, "Some practitioners seem to have no heart. . . . They seem to have their own agenda . . . maybe they're afraid to care." She believes that demonstrating care means being empathetic and being a "servant" in that the nurse "meets patients where *they* are." Catharine says that, "It's a very difficult place to be in when you serve somebody. You do something for somebody because they're at your table or in the hospital or because you're on that shift or because they call you on the phone. Then you care for them just because they happen to be there and you happen to be there and you just get to cut away the selfish attitude and you need to be able to effectively meet their needs." She believes that people have their own "inner wisdom" and that she "doesn't have all the answers."

Catharine demonstrates caring through observation, attending to patients' cues in how they look as well as how they say they feel. She uses communication and conveys to patients that she wants to help them maintain their dignity at all times. For example, she has realized that some people prefer to bathe themselves.

Catharine respects peoples' decisions to use any modality to heal themselves. She recognizes that many people use such treatments as herbs, homeopathy, and acupuncture, to name a few. She is not sure how or if she will integrate her education in traditional Chinese medicine with nursing. She does know that in her nursing phone work, she is constantly hearing patients cry out in frustration and confusion about such things as side effects of medications and not being touched by their health care practitioners. She says that it is "important to listen to people and not be on a different level." "I feel that nursing school added to my education and gave me the possibility of getting a job so that I could practice something. It gave me something but it didn't give me everything. Nurses need to have heart, too."

THERESE: SPECIALTY, NEONATAL INTENSIVE CARE (NICU)/INFEC-TIOUS DISEASE. Therese believes that she has demonstrated care in her nursing practice by encouraging people to "seek comfort, not just rid themselves of disease." She encourages people to learn to care for and nurture themselves. She gets "involved" with her patients so that she can help them help themselves. Therese says,

"Anyone can answer a question without really getting involved. I can't imagine doing that." In fact, the times Therese has gotten involved with her patients, especially the babies and families in the NICU, have been some of the most memorable times in her career. The "faith" that parents had in her care of their infant was "inspiring" to her.

Therese has used touch in her nursing practice with infants for many years. In her practice, she has always used massage and a type of light touch for premature babies that she now recognizes as being formalized in the practice known as therapeutic touch. Touch was very calming for babies. Addressing the patient's environment has also been a way that Therese has demonstrated care. She describes NICUs as "sterile, hostile environments that are often overstimulating to babies." She works with lowering noise and light levels to affect the babies' health. Environment is also a big issue for her work as a county infectious disease nurse. She stresses the importance of pure water and pure air to health and life. She encourages the use of water and interaction with nature to promote health. She is a "hot springs connoisseur."

Therese also demonstrates caring by discussing ways patients nurture themselves, such as with foods. She is asked a lot of questions about herbal medicine in her work as an infectious disease nurse. She has taken formal education in herbal medicine to answer some patient questions and has also developed a way to refer patients to get their questions answered when she cannot help. She believes that she demonstrates caring by helping her patients understand their bodies and any infectious disease they may have. She uses communication skills to build trust with patients. She believes that her "presence" and tone of voice are important to the development of a caring relationship.

Therese also demonstrates caring by being "sensitive." She gives the example of being present with a baby and being able to tailor her touch to the need of the baby so that it is not too stimulating and uncomfortable. She also prays for her "helpers" who are like guardian angels to give her strength and advice on how to help her patients.

LUKE: SPECIALTY, OUTPATIENT CARDIOPULMONARY REHABILITATION AND ICU. Luke says that demonstrating care means being nonjudgmental of patients. He has learned to provide nursing care in the "patient's own language." He asks the questions of patients that other caregivers might be afraid to ask, such as asking patients about their spirituality, their miracles, and their near-death experiences. Luke says that he is a "risk taker" and is not afraid to "be intimate with a patient" and be present for them to express their feelings. He also provides opportunities for his patients to "celebrate" and to cry when they need to. Luke has used touch, including massage and holding peoples' hands, when it is needed.

Demonstrating care for Luke means to provide a healing environment. He says, "You cannot isolate people from their environments and think that if you treat the individual and fit them back into their environment that they will heal." Luke invites family members to be with patients. He believes in being more flexible with organizational rules such as visiting hours so that patients' needs will be met. Luke also believes that the ICU environment is overstimulating and that patients end up "blocking out the experience because it is so overstimulating." Because of this, he demonstrates caring by adjusting lighting, monitoring odors, and using color, music, and live plants with patients.

In his work with the cardiopulmonary rehabilitation program, Luke uses nutrition as a caring modality. He uses massage, relaxation techniques, meditation, guided imagery, Chi Kung breathing exercises, and stretching in his care of patients. He plans to offer yoga in the near future. Patients choose what experiences they think will be helpful for their healing. For healing activities that are not provided by his office, Luke often accompanies his patients to the community facility that provides the activity. For example, one older patient was to go to an exercise class at a local recreation center. Luke went with him the first time so that he wouldn't have to go alone. Luke demonstrates care by being with the patient and walking with them through a difficult recovery time.

COMMON THEMES

The narratives from expert nurses, both retired and in practice, revealed several common themes regarding how nurses, despite their specialty area, demonstrate caring. For instance, the nurses all used touch as a way of demonstrating care. Touch was not always done in the same way; some did massages or back rubs whereas others held patients' hands. The nurses interviewed discussed some aspect of communication as a way of demonstrating care. Again, the manifestation of the type of communication technique was different from nurse to nurse, but the nurses all acknowledged communication as a way they have demonstrated care. Most of the nurses discussed the importance of nurses addressing the patient's environment as a way of demonstrating care. Because the nurses came from varied backgrounds, and some worked many years ago in health care environments that were very different from today, the issues regarding demonstrating care by addressing the patient's environment were very different. For example, one nurse working during the war was concerned about noise around the soldiers so that they would not be startled. She demonstrated caring by announcing herself when she walked into a room. Another nurse working in an ICU today addresses the noise issue in the patient's environment by dealing with the noise made by high-tech equipment. The ways the nurses address the environmental issues were somewhat different, but the nurse's ways of demonstrating care by addressing the environment was identified as fundamental to the process of building a healing relationship and demonstrating care.

All three of these areas—touch, communication, and environment—are key historical nursing fundamentals. It is not surprising that nurses spontaneously identified these fundamentals as being the framework wherein they demonstrate care.

The nurses were asked about two other general areas of nursing that appear in historical texts: nutrition and energy therapy. Most of the nurses agreed that addressing patient nutrition was included in their way of demonstrating care. Again, depending upon the work setting, the nurse had different ways of addressing the nutritional needs of patients. The NICU nurse works with babies who are breast-feeding or getting their feedings through a nasogastric tube. The cardiac rehab nurse teaches a "healthy heart diet" and the med-surg nurses sometimes spoonfeed water to patients who cannot take any other nourishment. The use of energy in nursing therapy was discussed by half of the nurses interviewed. In historical nursing texts, energy therapy is called "ray therapy" and usually refers to the use of the sun or an electromagnetic device for healing. "Energy therapy," a more encompassing term, is used here. The nurses with psychiatric experience described experiences they had with using electric shock and light therapies. Some of the older nurses remembered solar therapy being used for tuberculosis and other diseases. One of the younger nurses talked about the energy in her own body affecting the babies she works with in the NICU. Two of the nurses use therapeutic touch as a way of demonstrating care. Although nutrition and the use of energy were not mentioned as much as touch, environment, and communication, these two areas were indeed as fundamental to the experienced nurses' practice.

The five areas discussed in historical nursing texts were indeed the five areas discussed by the nurses in the interviews. A significant amount of variation and creativity was evident regarding how these five fundamentals were incorporated into patient care: Each nurse in practice addressed touch, communication, environment, nutrition, and energy. When the nurses were asked how they have demonstrated care throughout their career, they all had to stop and think. They began by talking about the type of patients they cared for or their work setting. It took more leading questions, such as, "How have you used the environment to demonstrate care, for example water, light, and sound?" to get the nurses to start pouring forth the numerous ways they have demonstrated care for patients. It seemed as if they really had never thought about the creative ways they had demonstrated care over the years.

Conclusion

Nurses demonstrate caring in so many simple ways every day, all day long, that it is second nature. It's so easy to get caught up in, and absorbed into, the more complex tasks of providing nursing care that many experienced nurses are not aware that they are the "embodied spirit of nursing" that Florence Nightingale outlined in her book, *Notes on Nursing*. This simple spirit of caring is demonstrated in many ways as the nurses in these narratives described. As nurses tell their stories, it is easy to see the treasure-house of knowledge in the caring profession of nursing. Nurses must tell their stories and talk about the ways they demonstrate caring, just as other professions discuss the ways they fulfill their missions.

From historical writings, as well as from present-day nurses' narratives, five fundamental areas can be identified as nurses' areas of expertise. This is not to say that other healing professions do not address these areas of healing. It is to say that as our colleagues in the medical field, for example, identify medicine and surgery as their areas of expertise, nurses can embrace the five fundamentals of caring: touch, communication, environment, nutrition, and energy as the areas they specialize in when delivering care. We can become experts in the research and development of caring modalities that address the needs of the patient in these five areas. Part Three addresses these five fundamental areas and some of the more specific ways nurses employ these caring modalities in their practice.

References

Astrom, G., Norberg, A., & Hallberg, I. (1995). Skilled nurses' experience of caring. *Journal of Professional Nursing, 11* (2), 110–118.

Donahue, M. (1996). *Nursing: The finest art* (2nd ed.). St. Louis, MO: Mosby–Yearbook, Inc.

Frank, S. C. M. (1959). *Foundations of nursing* (2nd ed.). Philadelphia: W.B. Saunders Co.

Harmer, B. (1924). *Text-book of the principles and practice of nursing.* New York: Macmillan Co.

Micozzi, M. (1996). *Fundamentals of complementary and alternative medicine.* New York: Churchill Livingstone Inc.

Nightingale, F. (1957). *Notes on nursing.* Philadelphia, PA: J.B. Lippincott Co.

Taber's cyclopedic medical dictionary (18th ed.). (1997). Philadelphia: F.A. Davis Company.

Tracy, M. (1938). *Nursing: An art and a science.* St. Louis, MO: C.V. Mosby Co.

Webster's new collegiate dictionary (1956). (2nd ed.) Springfield, MA: G. & C. Merriam Co.

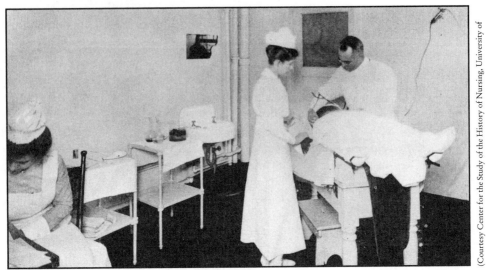

The subtleties of care

All our architects of fate working in these walls of time,

Some with massive deeds and great, Some with ornaments of rhyme.

Nothing useless is or low, Each thing in its place is best.

And what seems but idle show, Strengthens and supports the rest.

For the structure that we raise, Time is with materials filled.

Our todays and yesterdays are the blocks with which we build.

Truly shape and fashion these, Leave no yawning gaps between.

Think not because no man sees, Such things will remain unseen.

—HENRY WADSWORTH LONGFELLOW

CHAPTER 5

Envisioning the Future of Caring

How nurses have demonstrated caring to patients has evolved over the years. With the exception of the technological advances in health care and their impact on nursing care, patients' needs for caring nurses have gone unchanged. The need for care in a biomedical world has actually increased. There are constant "threads" of how nurses have demonstrated caring throughout history, such as holding a hand, being *present* while listening to patients' concerns, and providing a healing environment. The public expects these caring acts from nurses.

Nurses are at a crossroads where decisions about the future of nursing practice must be made, while taking into consideration the needs and expectations of the public as well as the expectations of a changing health care environment in chaos. As a number of the nurses' narratives in Chapter 4 described, it is often difficult for the creative and intelligent nurse to work in an environment that does not support, let alone encourage, a caring practice. Many nurses, such as Catharine and Luke, made decisions to leave hospital practice to seek out alternative environments more supportive of caring practice. Nurses who have become specialized in a particular caring modality, such as massage, must often open private practices to do their work because they are unable to integrate these caring modalities into the nursing care they give in the hospital or home health settings. Often, they are not given the time or the support of administrators to do so.

It is very difficult in many fast-paced health care settings to provide caring therapies. Nurses must often delegate these interventions to unlicensed caregivers. For example, nurses no longer routinely provide back care, AM care, or PM care to patients.

These skills are seen as chores to be delegated to nursing assistants. Nurses have also watched as other disciplines, such as physical therapy, provide the caring therapies they no longer provide. In her narrative, Joan mentioned that she learned the Sister Kenny method of hydrotherapies with its wraps and packs. This caring modality was successfully used in nursing practice in the care for polio victims. Now, it is rare that a nurse has knowledge of this type of historical treatment. Physical therapists in hospitals do use hydrotherapies, as well as hot and cold applications or packs for patient rehabilitation, but it is rare that these hydrotherapy services are used for healing patients with disease. Chapter 8 discusses hydrotherapy in greater detail.

A similar situation exists for the nutrition services provided to patients. Nurses in some hospitals rarely see the tray of food the patient receives, let alone help the patient choose appropriate foods that promote healing. When I was a nursing student, I worked on a surgical ward where I cared for a patient who had had minor surgery the previous day and was allowed a regular diet by the surgeon, but she had a very weak appetite. Her lunch tray came to her room with beef bourguignonne on her plate. I saw her turn green at the sight of it. Her body said "no" to the food, but she seemed confused about whether or not she should eat what had been given to her. It is not uncommon for people going through unusual situations, such as surgery, to be confused about how and what to eat. My role at that time was to help her choose food that would be nourishing. Nurses often demonstrate caring by providing this type of guidance to patients during a health crisis.

If nurses continue the trend of being involved only in the technical care of patients and allowing other disciplines to take responsibility for some of the fundamental caring opportunities, such as providing nourishment, physical treatments, and comfort, nurses may lose their ability to provide holistic and integrative care. Will nurses be able to find ways to provide total patient care? If the role of the nurse does not include these foundational caring behaviors, will nurses still be perceived as demonstrating caring? Is the reason we are viewed by the public as a caring profession because we attend to the day-to-day holistic needs of patients? Nurses are faced with many professional choices. Nurses are choosing how to provide technical care and they are choosing how to provide caring modalities. Nurses are also choosing how to integrate the two.

Must nurses who want to focus on the caring aspects of nursing relinquish their interests and skills to the more technical aspects of nursing? Where will a nurse who wants to integrate both biomedical and caring skills practice? These are just some of the questions and challenges nurses, nurse-educators, and nursing leaders are encountering at the crossroads. It is also these types of concerns that, if left unresolved, can lead to crisis.

Avoiding a Caregiver's Crisis

Part of the practice of integrative nursing is the ability to create a way to provide both biomedical skills and caring modalities to patients. In looking at the future and how nurses will demonstrate caring, a climate of uncertainty exists around the concept of integrative nursing. Even though it may not have been called integrative nursing, many nurses and administrators have been seeking ways to meet both the biomedical and caring needs of the patients in an integrated approach. It is a difficult question for some, one that often gets swept aside because the issue has not reached "crisis" proportions.

Crises occur when people's coping mechanisms no longer work. Crises can take many forms. From a caring perspective, a crisis in nursing occurs when nurses are not able to provide or demonstrate caring. I have seen nurses work with patients and not demonstrate caring. I have heard patients talk about this occurring to them. So I am aware that this crisis can happen to any of us for many reasons, both personal and professional. It has happened to me as well.

When I divorced my first husband I experienced tremendous sorrow even though the divorce was a good decision for me. I was unable to be "present" with my patients because I was so preoccupied with my own sadness. At the time I was providing reflexology and other complementary therapy services to patients. After discussing the situation with my medical director, I decided that the most caring thing for my patients and for me was not to practice for a few weeks. I was unable to care for my patients and I knew it. I also knew that it would not be forever. It was a shocking moment when I realized that I could not care for patients the way they needed me to. Some might say that it was indeed a caring act for me to *not* try to demonstrate caring for my patients. I have met nurses who have left the profession at the point where they could no longer care. This was not an option for me. From that experience I learned a little more about my humanity and I thanked my patients and my nursing work for showing it to me.

I have also been in the situation where a nursing director refused to allow me to provide the level of caring service I wanted to provide . . . at least on work time. I had a ninety-five-year-old patient who was in a wheelchair but was still able to provide community service by teaching preschool teachers. Because she had done this often, without charge, I thought it only appropriate that she receive professional services for a nominal charge. I assisted her once a week with her bath and massage. Because of her culture and upbringing, she talked about really valuing the health benefits of bath and massage. One day my director said that I could no longer provide these services to her and that the care would be delegated to unlicensed caregivers. It was an "executive" decision over which I had no control. This perceived lack of control over my practice seemed like a crisis. I decided to continue to provide the service for this patient, on my own time. In this case the crisis of my inability to demonstrate care (as part of my job) was being directed from an outside source. Nurses can feel a sense of crisis when outer or inner circumstances make it difficult to provide the necessary care.

Crises are intrinsic to life as well as nursing practice and care. It is what we do with the crisis in the moment that determines the future. Each individual nursing decision defines the future of nursing practice and how the public perceives our profession. The Chinese word for crisis is made up of two characters—one meaning danger and

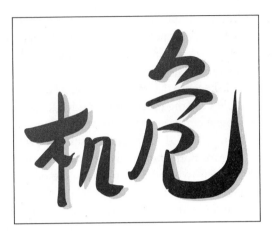

FIGURE 5-1
The Chinese character for crisis

the other meaning opportunity (see Figure 5–1). Based on the Chinese definition, within the crisis and danger of not being able to demonstrate care for patients, is also our opportunity to make caring happen.

Nursing is at a crossroads. It offers many possibilities and opportunities to endure a caregiver's crisis and continue to grow as a caring profession. Although I have experienced this challenge many times, it is not my intention to provide the *answers* about the future of nurses demonstrating care. That will be determined by all of us in the day-to-day decisions we make. From a historical perspective, it seems that the practice of professional nursing has evolved to the point where it no longer necessarily includes the fundamental caring practices of touch, environment, nutrition, communication, and use of energy. One of the purposes of exploring one's history, either personally or professionally, is to seek understanding or connection with one's identity. In seeking to understand nursing history, we can see threads of nursing identity in how we demonstrate caring, especially in these five fundamental areas. In addition to gaining understanding, another purpose of exploring history is to be able to look at trends in history and provide insight into the future based upon those trends. The future of professional nursing may not include caring modalities, and professional nurses may not be paid to provide excellent caring service. Instead, the nurse's technical skills may be valued above all else. Nurses must recognize their frustrations with the limitations on caring practice as an emotional wake up call, an indication of the need to practice nursing from a more integrative approach that values biomedical and caring skills equally. Nurses have the ability to navigate through a caregiver's crisis.

Navigation through anything, including a crisis, takes thought and preparation. Just as caring for a single patient takes a plan of care, so does planning and caring for the future of nursing practice. All plans can be flexible. There are many routes to reaching a goal. The plan is not the goal; it is a representation of the process of achieving one's goals. The plan evolves as it emerges from within, which in this case would be from within each nurse. Many nurses have chosen to use reflection in clinical decision making. Reflection can also be used to get in touch with the "inner" navigator who can help us through any crisis or health care challenge.

Reflections on the Future of Caring Practice

The remainder of this chapter offers you the opportunity to *reflect* on some of the important questions you will need to address when navigating the choices of direction for the future of your caring career as well as the future of the nursing profession as a whole. There are five reflections. You may want to have a notebook or journal with you as you ponder the questions in each reflection.

REFLECTION 1: BELIEFS AND PARADIGMS

What are the beliefs, values, and paradigms upon which I make choices about how I care for patients? What are they now and what might they be in the future?

NURSING CULTURE.   Historically, most nurses have received the bulk of their clinical education in hospitals. As discussed in Chapter 1, most nurses today are fully educated in the biomedical model of health care and receive much of their experience in a biomedical facility such as a hospital or outpatient facility. Nursing culture has become identified with that of biomedicine. Nurses of the future will make choices about whether or not to be educated in hospitals. Our decisions about nursing care in the present will affect the relationship between nursing and the biomedical world.

The variety of ways nurses have been educated and have practiced throughout history, including biomedical training, have created a nursing *culture.* Cultures change and evolve and are the creation of the people who make them up. Health care culture is changing and so is nursing culture. When nurses enter into a relationship with a patient they bring their personal as well as professional culture with them. There are many patients who do not know anything about the language, health beliefs, values, and practices of nursing culture. For some patients, entering a hospital or even the care of a nurse is similar to going to another country.

> **QUESTION:** How do I care for a "foreigner" in "my country"?
> **QUESTION:** How do I feel about providing care for a patient in his home or in a facility other than a hospital?
> **QUESTION:** What will the future of the hospital be and what role might I take in the development of hospital care?

Many nurses, including Florence Nightingale, have held a vision of nursing care that is separate from hospital care. Nightingale said, "We are still on the threshold of nursing. In the future, may a better way be opened! May the methods by which every infant, every human being will have the best chance of health, the methods by which every sick person will have the best chance of recovery, be learned and practiced! Hospitals are only an intermediate state of civilization never intended, at all events, to take in the whole sick population" (Donahue, 1996, p. 417).

HEALTH BELIEF SYSTEMS. Many cultures have highly developed health belief and health care systems. The Asian and Native American systems are thousands of years old and have served people quite well up to and beyond the advent of bio-medicine. Nurses are continuously exposed to a wealth of various health beliefs and practices by working so closely with people. As we get to know our patients and develop a respectful, caring relationship with them we learn about their values and beliefs which may differ from our own personal and/or professional culture.

As a rule the biomedical culture does not embrace ethnic and cultural differences in the health arena. "In keeping with the scientific tradition, modern biomedicine has striven to separate itself from broader cultural concerns and influences (and has considered itself largely successful in the attempt). It has excluded religious, metaphysical, and philosophical considerations from its explanatory models of disease and dysfunction. It has claimed for itself a unique value-neutrality and (ironically) valued that neutrality as good" (O'Connor, 1995, p. 22). Nursing culture is very different. Because of the focus on creating healing relationships with people, nurses continually interact with cultures and individuals with varying health beliefs.

QUESTION: What are my personal/professional health beliefs and how are they similar and different?

QUESTION: What are the health beliefs and values of my patients?

QUESTION: Should nursing culture reflect the health beliefs and values of the biomedical culture in the future?

QUESTION: How do my health beliefs and those of my patients affect my ability to effectively demonstrate caring?

HEALTH CARE PARADIGMS. Biomedical culture has traditionally been disease-oriented as opposed to wellness-oriented. The majority of the health care dollars in the United States are spent on identifying the cause of disease and creating a way of killing or disabling the disease process. Disease is considered "bad" and "abnormal" and the absence of disease, or at least the appearance of the absence of disease, is desirable and highly valued. The paradigm or thought pattern surrounding the health care industry and those involved in supporting the biomedical worldview is based upon this desire for and belief in a disease-free, normal state. This paradigm has manifested as the "fight" against disease and the plethora of antitreatments: antivirals, antibacterials, antibiotics, antifungals, antidotes, anticoagulants, anticholinergics, antidiuretics, anti-inflammatories, antigens, and antiseptics, to name a few. Those who hold a disease-oriented paradigm often compare the body to a machine that can be controlled and/or repaired. One author, Joan Engebretson, calls this paradigm the "mechanical explanatory" paradigm (1998, p. 39). Engebretson also discusses three other paradigms that have defined health care. The "purification paradigm" originated with the Egyptians. "Purification and the avoidance of pollution are the purposes of many healing activities that operate on the physical and symbolic levels" (p. 39). The "balance paradigm" is manifested in many Asian healing systems as well as in Hippocratic medicine. As discussed previously, this paradigm of balance of such concepts as hot and cold has been part of the nursing paradigm as well. The fourth paradigm, "supranormal, follows the magical/religious ideology in which illness is related to the breech of a taboo or a lack of integrity with higher powers" (p. 39).

QUESTION: What is my paradigm or worldview about health and healing? Can I hold more than one worldview? Does it ever change?

QUESTION: How does my paradigm affect my nursing practice and how I demonstrate caring?

REFLECTION 2: PRACTICING INTEGRATIVE NURSING

How can I create a practice that is integrative in that I:

- Effectively and creatively integrate my biomedical and caregiving skills?
- Have the time to evaluate patient need for comfort, balance, and homeostasis and "put the patient in the best possible condition for nature to work upon him"?
- Observe and act upon the holistic needs of patients?

Throughout history, nursing practice has developed side by side with medicine. Nurses have worked in and supported the biomedical worldview. Yet throughout history nurses have also tried to answer the question, "How am I, as a *nurse,* to *be* with my patients"? Florence Nightingale, one of the early leaders of nursing, showed us the fundamentals of caring for patients and identifying what *being* a nurse is all about. She considered nursing to be the "finest of fine arts" (Donahue, 1996, p. ix). Defining nursing as an art implies that providing nursing care and demonstrating caring to others is a creative act. For nurses to integrate biomedical and caring skills, as well as provide holistic care, they are faced with the challenge of creating their practice.

Many early nurses were members of religious orders that gave guidance on how to care for patients. The care given was to address the spiritual needs of the patient as a matter of course rather than choice. Patients expected nurses to provide religious guidance during their time of need because the nurses were of the religious orders. Nurses today do not have these kinds of affiliations. The guidelines for practice are usually evidenced through administrative policy and procedure manuals. The manuals represent the *task* part of what we do, but not the *spirit* of what we do with patients, nor does it, or can it, tell us the *effort,* or how we do the tasks we do every day. The spirit and effort we put into our work are uniquely ours. It is what makes our care special to others and to ourselves. That spirit of creativity is what generates the interest and the energy to demonstrate caring.

Nurses from religious orders had a calling. Nurses, such as Nightingale, who practiced during wartime, had a calling. What is our calling now? Why should we be creative and put forth an effort to care for others? Having talked with a number of nurses about how they are creative in the ways they demonstrate caring to others, I found that each one is creative in her own way and her motivation for being creative and caring is unique. I also found that each nurse has a personal vision of what caring is about. Barbara, Anne, Therese, Luke, and Catharine were not wartime nurses, but they have a vision of why and how they care. They demonstrate that, "Nursing is not merely a technique but a process that incorporates the elements of soul, mind and imagination. Its essence lies in the creative imagination, the sensitive spirit, and the intelligent understanding that provide the very foundation for effective nursing care" (Donahue, 1996, p. ix).

QUESTION: How am I creative in my practice?

THE COURAGE TO CREATE/THE COURAGE TO INTEGRATE.   It takes courage to be creative. Many say that creativity takes time so they focus on the quicker way of doing things the way "they have always been done." Some people do not like to be creative, they do not like to try new things. That's okay. It does take courage and an element of risk to be creative. Being creative means being a leader even if you are only a leader of one, yourself.

Integrating caring and biomedical skills takes creativity. There's no road map. Being holistic and addressing the individual needs of a patient takes creativity. Helping a patient achieve greater balance and comfort takes creativity. Nurses are courageous when they embrace creativity in themselves, in their patients, and in each other. Nurses who seek ways to maintain a connection with fundamental nursing modalities for use in practice will need the courage to create a new practice.

How nursing is practiced is a reflection of the type of society we live in. Nursing care is part of the culture of a society. As members of society, nurses help create that society and a history by thoughts and daily actions. If nurses choose not to change they are still creating history and influencing society. All manifestations of art and creativity are linked to the history of various cultures. Rollo May writes, "If you wish to understand the psychological and spiritual temper of any historical period, you can do no better than to look long and searchingly at its art. . . . Creativity must be seen in the work of the scientist as well as in that of the artist, in the thinker as well as in the aesthetician; and one must not rule out the extent to which it is present in captains of modern technology. Creativity as Webster's rightly indicates, is basically the process of *making, of bringing into being*" (May, 1994, pp. 40, 52). Nursing history is steeped with art, innovative thinking, and creativity.

The reason creativity takes courage is that in each creative act and each attempt to try something new, there is an inherent sense of letting go of the "old way." This letting go does not have to be a complete erasing of history, personally or professionally. Integration implies the possibility of creating by "adding to" not necessarily "taking away." People often think that to create something new or to change they must "give up" or "destroy" the old. I saw this demonstrated years ago when I participated in a game at a public health conference I attended.

The group leader had everyone stand up and face a partner. We were given two minutes to look at our partner and take in the details of what they looked like. Then we had to turn our backs to each other and "*change* our appearance in five different ways." Everyone in the group *removed* five things from their appearance. Of course, the leader showed us through this exercise that to all of us, over one hundred people, *change* had meant to *remove,* or *give up.* He also pointed out that very often this is the prevailing perception of change in businesses and health care. He then asked us to try changing our appearance by "adding to" or "rearranging." There was an audible sigh of relief throughout the conference hall because people are often uncomfortable about change if it means having to "give up."

Nurses often react to the impulse to change with the same hesitation. Creativity is often linked with the notion of change, and change with removal. We forget that sometimes to change, we simply need to *add.* The concept of change as removal or letting go can be threatening to our sense of self. It is a natural reaction. Change as an "addition" to does not create the same response.

Being creative is an expression of self. It's sometimes a risky part of being who we are. Leah Curtin, editor of *Nursing Management,* wrote an intriguing editorial where she compared the concept of the nursing *team* to the flock of seagulls in the book, *Jonathan Livingston Seagull.* She writes about Jonathan's absolute love of flying. He was compelled by his search for excellence in flying and found that because of this he was cast out by the other gulls in his flock. Curtin compares the story of Jonathan Livingston Seagull to nursing teams. She writes, "Jonathan's problem was that he loved to fly. . . . He wasn't trying to stand out among the gulls. He didn't want power in the flock. . . . Teams as they are generally found in business and health care today penalize creativity, punish dissent and promote mediocrity. . . . Love for the work has nothing to do with team membership. The law of the flock rules, and woe be unto any who stand out. Any creative sparks are snuffed out in meetings as flock members waste time with screeing around the issues, fighting over fish heads and preening their feathers in public" (1998, p. 5).

It takes courage, passion, and a love for what we do to be creative. Being creative and integrative can be energizing. The future of nursing will be an expression of the integration of all that we know and have learned about caring for others. Nurses need not ever feel ashamed or be shamed about providing care that, although seemingly simple, such as a mother caring for a child, has historically been an effective means of caring. Nor should the nurse feel ashamed, or be shamed, for the decision to demonstrate caring through the use of science and technology. The integration process, the way we choose to comfort, and the demonstration of a holistic caring process, will be borne of our relationships with patients. It will be borne of our lived experience as caregivers and our courage to be who we are as human beings who just happen to be nurses.

QUESTION: How do I feel about change?
QUESTION: How have I had the courage to create?
QUESTION: What is my role in the "flock"?

REFLECTION 3: WHO PERFORMS THE FUNDAMENTALS?

In the future, who will perform the fundamentals of nursing care, e.g., the bathing, the back rubs, the feeding, the listening? Nursing textbooks from the late 1800s and early 1900s clearly show that the fundamentals of nursing have long been considered important aspects of health care. The tasks involved in bedside nursing occupy the entire text. Professional nursing is equated with providing good bedside nursing. Today, the skills of bedside nursing are often delegated to unlicensed assistant personnel (UAP). It is considered more cost effective and often viewed as a better use of the professional nurse's time to delegate these duties. But as was so often mentioned in the nurses' narratives in Chapter 4, the nurse who delegates these duties often does not achieve the same level of rapport or relationship with the patient that she is able to when she is providing the intimate bedside care herself.

There are other historical changes that have occurred as well. Nurses rarely have patients in the hospital who are recuperating. Most are acutely ill and require a different type of bedside care. The home care nurse rarely provides basic nursing care. Usually a home health aide does that work when the professional nurse is not present. Who will perform these fundamental nursing tasks in the future? If patients expect the nurse to provide the care, and one of nursing's slogans is "Every patient deserves a nurse," why aren't professional nurses providing the care?

Our history shows the fundamentals of nursing care as being of tremendous value to the outcome of patient care. Will the nursing research of the future support this value and tradition? Will nurses continue the trend of moving away from the fundamentals of baths, feeding, back rubs, and talking with patients? Will educators continue to teach the fundamentals to professional nursing students or will that be left to the nursing assistant programs? These are all questions that will continue to be addressed because nurses still value the fundamentals of care.

Throughout the history of nursing there have been attempts to provide the opportunity for the patient to receive all care from a professional nurse, if the nurse chooses to do so. This model of nursing care is called "total patient care" and means that the professional nurse provides total care for the patient; there are no nursing assistants. Another similar model, called "primary nursing," allows the nurse to choose whether or not to delegate the fundamental care of the patient to an assistant. These models have been practiced in inpatient and outpatient settings.

In the journal article, "Sources of Satisfaction in Hospital Nursing Practice," the authors discuss primary nursing. "While the pressures of shorter lengths of stay and reduced staffing may create a tendency toward a more fragmented, functional approach to care delivery, continuity in nurses' patient assignments has been shown to be strongly related to perceived job significance and identity. Primary nursing is the delivery method that provides continuity and identifies accountability for nursing outcomes" (Tonges, Rothstein, & Carter, 1998, p. 60). The study discussed in this article found that ". . . it is very important to staff's well-being that we hold to our basic values as reflected in continuity of nurse-patient relationships, authority to initiate independent nursing actions, individual accountability for clinical outcomes and regular feedback from managers" (p. 60). It is possible for nurses to have greater accountability and authority for patient care. Throughout history there have been numerous examples of nursing leaders who have done just that.

> **QUESTION:** How can I draw upon historical experiences to reestablish my connection with the fundamentals of nursing care? Do I want to practice nursing fundamentals?
>
> **QUESTION:** Who will bathe, massage, walk, feed, position, and talk with patients?
>
> **QUESTION:** How do I feel about having responsibility and authority for patient care? Will this affect the way I develop healing relationships?

MODELS FOR CARING PRACTICE.   One historical example of nurses having authority and responsibility for their practice can be found in the work of Lydia Hall. Hall practiced nursing in the 1950s and 1960s. She developed the Loeb Center for Nursing and Rehabilitation in New York. Hall saw the nurse's role as one of comforter and more. According to Hall, the professional nurse was able to offer the patient a learning experience as well as a comforting one. Hall called this "nurturing." The nurturer was someone who "fosters learning, someone who fosters growing up emotionally, someone who even fosters healing" (Hall, 1969, p. 86). Hall did not believe that the nursing care of a patient should be left to practical nurses and aides at a time when the patient was in the most teachable state, during rehabilitation and recovery.

At the Loeb Center, nurses were not "practical doctors" with the goal of curing patients. Nurses were autonomous and practiced caring. Physicians were consultants to the nurses. And remarkably, the Loeb Center was a success. Nurses were on waiting lists to work there. Patients and physicians were very happy with the care provided. The Loeb Center provided a unique, creative alternative to the "progressive" care of the time. "Progressive patient care implies that, as the patient needs less medical care, he needs not only more nursing care, but more professional nursing care and teaching" (Hall, 1963, p. 806). Hall developed her practice based on the belief that, "Bodily care of an intimate nature has long been recognized as belonging to nurses. Bathing, feeding, toileting, dressing, undressing, positioning and moving, as well as maintaining a healthful environment, are encompassed in the area of bodily care expertness" (Loose, 1994, p. 174).

Lydia Hall was correct that many of the fundamentals, caring nursing activities done with patients, are very intimate. Are nurses who are not thoroughly educated and experienced in these fundamentals willing and able to explore the intimate relationship with a patient so often encountered in professional nursing? How does a nurse know how close is "too close" when interacting with a patient? How intimate and close to patients will the nurses of the future be?

INTIMACY.   Carol Montgomery writes that "caring has been viewed as dangerous for the one caring, such that caregivers are urged not to care too much, for fear of burnout" (1996, p. 52). In her narrative, Joan said that she was told not to cry with a family because it was not "professional." Crying with a patient or their family meant that the nurse was "too" involved. How close can a professional nurse get without getting burned out? How can a nurse balance the care she provides with protection from overinvolvement? When is a nurse "overcaring"?

Montgomery writes that "rather than trying to resolve the paradox of how close is too close, an alternative . . . is to look at the nature of the connection itself. There is a distinct qualitative difference between helping relationships connected at the level of the ego and those connected at the level of something greater. The individuals involved in a caring encounter experience their common substance at the level of their shared humanity or spirit. In contrast, what we usually refer to as 'overinvolvement' is characterized by a highly personalized connection that is not experienced in this larger sense" (1996, p. 54). She identifies ego-based relationships as those in which the nurse is attempting to fix or cure. This fix or cure model can be a barrier to the creation of healing relationships. Many nurses have concerns about the issue of professional boundaries and how the concept fits with their value of creating healing relationships.

Nurses know that being intimate with patients, drawing forth that common thread of humanity between the hearts of those engaged in a healing relationship, can be energizing and uplifting for those involved. The nurse learns in the process of developing a healing relationship what such a relationship is like. For example, I once shed tears with a parent whose infant had died. This parent told me later that seeing my tears was helpful for him. It gave him reassurance that crying was "okay." I did not cry so much that I was unable to provide care for him. The tears were the caring "modality" with this parent. When professional boundaries are relaxed too much the nurse becomes ineffective at providing care. If the nurse places herself in this position often, she may start to experience overcare, energy drain, and burnout.

QUESTION: What is it like when I am energized by caring for a patient?

QUESTION: How have I experienced the common humanity or spirit between myself and a patient? What did I learn from that experience?

QUESTION: Has there been a time when I experienced an energy drain from caring for a patient? If so, how might I have allowed my desire for cure and my ego direct the relationship rather than allowing the patient's experience to be his own?

QUESTION: What type of model of caring practice (such as the Loeb Center) might be helpful for me as I make decisions about the future of my practice?

REFLECTION 4: HAVE I BECOME DEPENDENT ON THE BIOMEDICAL WORLD?

In what ways have I come to depend on the biomedical world? What would I do if biomedicine as I know it (e.g., drugs and surgeries) became unavailable for me, my family, and/or my patients? Could I still practice as a nurse?

As has been discussed throughout this book, nurses have been invested in the biomedical model of care for a number of years. Nurses are also aware that many people lack access to the biomedical health care system because it is often too expensive. The growing cost of health care is overwhelming for the average citizen of most nations. An article in *Modern Healthcare* states that "personal and national wealth often set the threshold for access to care. But social policy, health care payment systems and cultural factors also bear heavily on the utilization of medical technology. New technology has increased healthcare spending worldwide despite advocates' claims that technology ultimately saves money. Clinicians' swelling toolboxes—and the extent to which governments try to control their contents—significantly shape utilization worldwide" (Hensley, 1998, p. 24). "Japan and the U.S. are neck-and-neck for leadership in drug consumption. In 1997, each American consumed drugs costing $379 while a typical Japanese used $373 worth, according to IMS health. . . . Searching for a quick fix to their health problems, Americans have long been known as pill-poppers" (p. 25).

Nurses who work in large urban hospitals may find it easier to address patient demand for "quick fixes and pills." But as any senior nurse or rural health nurse can relay, quick fixes and expensive drugs, assessment devices, and interventions are not available to large populations in most countries.

THE LESSONS OF RURAL NURSING. I worked in rural Montana for six years and found that the culture and the economy, as well as the land and climate, frequently dictated health care decisions. Working in a small log cabin with the nearest small hospital forty-five minutes away, and the nearest trauma center two hours away, meant that we often provided nursing care that was very different from what I learned during my nursing education in Los Angeles. I was aware of the expense of every 2" × 2" gauze pad. The latest antibiotics were not always available at the small pharmacy nearby, which was closed for business on the weekends. Getting a quick CBC was impossible. Our labs were picked up by the mailman during the week and sent to a lab two hours away. We had no x-ray equipment.

We performed a lot of first aid and we had an ambulance with a trained staff of nurses and emergency medical technicians. We practiced the fundamentals of nursing, suggested dietary changes when needed, and provided comfort and pain relief often without narcotics. We assessed and planned care with patients based on their economic realities, health and cultural beliefs, and the health care options available in their rural community. As any nurse who has worked in public or rural health knows, the relationships with patients in rural settings are very different from those in the hospital setting. The relationships formed with these patients, although very rich, are in many ways more challenging.

I learned how much I had to offer a community as a nurse when I worked in Montana. I didn't always have the option of letting the biomedical world perform its magic; my patients didn't either. But it was really okay. In fact, I developed a deep respect and gratitude for the biomedical health system with all its sterilized gauze, throw away instruments, and miracle drugs. I also developed a deep respect for caring and nursing science, which enabled me to help many patients through some challenging times without the aide of biomedicine.

> **QUESTION:** What would nursing practice be like without the technology and practices of the biomedical world?
>
> **QUESTION:** What types of modalities would I use in practice if my practice did not include assisting patients with pharmaceutical drugs and surgeries?

REFLECTION 5: ADDRESSING THE PATIENT'S GROWING NEED FOR COMFORT AND STRESS REDUCTION

How will I address the patients' growing need for comfort and stress reduction? What modalities will I use and how will I honor patients' requests for specific caring modalities?

In Agatha's narrative in Chapter 4, she discusses her desire to help a patient who is recovering from surgery. The patient is complaining of pain yet the patient has all the symptoms of exposure to narcotics. The patient has a very low respiratory rate and pinpoint pupils. Because Agatha has given the patient all the narcotics she can safely have, Agatha looks for other ways to comfort the patient. She also discusses her concern that "more and more patients" seem to need more and more narcotics for pain relief.

How does Agatha honor her patients' requests for pain relief when she has used the limit of narcotics? Are their other modalities that nurses could use in the PACUs to address pain issues? These are the very questions that led me to the exploration of what nurses have done throughout history to demonstrate caring and address the comfort needs of patients. Nurses in many developed countries no longer utilize historical comfort measures, nor are they taught these measures in schools of nursing. Yet there are many patients who continue to request modalities for comfort and cure, no longer available in many nursing services, that they believe will help their healing process. Many of these therapies are now called alternative and complementary therapies and are practiced by lay practitioners who specialize in a particular modality.

> **QUESTION:** How do I react when a patient asks me to call their acupuncturist to come to the hospital to give them a treatment for their nausea? What would I do if they took a homeopathic or herbal remedy for nausea instead of asking me for some antiemetic drug? How would I feel if they told me that they didn't want medicine and that they knew that by putting a cool cloth on their forehead they would feel less nauseated?

> **QUESTION:** How do I honor patients' ways of dealing with their nausea or any other condition?

HONORING PATIENTS.   When nurses honor patients they bestow reverence upon them. Honoring a patient is about demonstrating respect for a patient's choices in dealing with their health or lack of health. Honoring a patient is more than tolerating the different ways he chooses to experience healing. Honoring a patient means being acutely aware of the patient's accountability and choices in healing as his own creative process. Honoring a patient's wishes for care means honoring the spirit that helped him make the choice, the same spirit that can choose drugs and surgeries as a modality as well. When nurses dishonor the spirit of choice in the patient, the patient will often turn away. Patients are often aware of when a health practitioner dishonors them and their choices for care, even if the practitioner says nothing. Patients can be quite astute at reading a practitioner's nonverbal cues.

Many people continue to use some form of complementary therapy in addition to using the modalities offered by biomedical practitioners. The emergence of this phenomenon will be discussed in greater detail in Chapter 6. The public's use of such therapies is responsible for much of the paradigm shift in many Western nations to the increased use of complementary therapies by mainstream practitioners. Dr. Jeanne Achterberg writes, "Paradigm shifts are precipitated by crises." She says that, "The crisis that will precipitate a paradigm shift, a revolution in the linear and constrained view of reality, is and is not about medicine or health care as we know it. It is not about science. It is not about financial exigencies that have shaken health consumers and care givers out of any complacency that modern health care would be delivered for every need or proffer a right and prosperous livelihood. It is and is not about a crisis in a technology that failed to eradicate the problems of the civilized world. Fundamentally, it is a crisis in human values, of how we regard and care for one another, ourselves, and all things alive and nonorganic in our world" (Achterberg, 1998, p. 62).

CHOOSING MODALITIES.   Nursing as a caring profession can endure as long as it is not married to the concept of providing only the modalities acceptable to the biomedical world or culture. Our work is with the patient. Our focus is the patient and honoring his needs and decisions. "Many patients are using multiple modalities of healing. Biomedicine with its scientific-positivist base has made great advances in the treatment of disease. However, the lay public's search for alternative modalities may be related to a search for meaning and recognition of aspects of life beyond the material. Practitioners incorporating multiple modalities provide a model for integrated practice and are able to meet patient needs and preferences in using more avenues to promote client health" (Engebretson, 1998, p. 42). It is not too late for nurses to again embrace the wealth of modalities they have offered patients throughout history, expanding their repertoire of ways to demonstrate caring. Patients are looking for the full "meal," not just the appetizer or dessert. Nurses have much to offer patients in their search for meaning because we see so much of life at a time when "meaning" is so critical. We are also a profession that has extensive firsthand knowledge of the complementary therapies sought by the public.

Dr. Achterberg writes, "A significant body of evidence suggests that an imminent change in the way health care is delivered is on the horizon, and that movement in complementary and alternative medicine appears to be the provocateur—quite independent of research, efficacy, economics or legislation" (1998, p. 66). In looking to the future of nursing practice, it is imperative that we recognize the public's continued interest in complementary therapies and what these therapies represent to them and to ourselves.

> **QUESTION:** How do I feel about complementary therapies? How much do I know about them and how might I already be using them in practice?

Conclusion

Nurses have been practicing complementary therapies throughout history. Embracing the concept of meeting public need for complementary therapies doesn't necessarily mean that nurses have to do anything different. It does mean that we may need to reevaluate any emphasis we may have placed on the biomedical aspects of nursing and find a better way to create a balance between our new scientific findings and some of the historic and time-proven caring modalities. The following chapters explore the link between demonstrating care using some of the complementary therapies of today and demonstrating care using the fundamentals of nursing found in historical nursing texts. It is exciting to think that as nurses realize the opportunity to reclaim their history in the use of caring fundamentals, and use them in new ways to enhance the science and art of nursing practice, they might also be in a position to better meet the needs of patients for a healing relationship that includes complementary therapies.

References

Achterberg, J. (1998). Between the lightning and thunder: The pause before the shifting paradigm. *Alternative Therapies, 4* (3), 62–66.

Curtain, L. (1998). Jonathan Livingston Seagull on teams. *Nursing Management, 29* (1), 5–6.

Donahue, M. P. (1996). *Nursing: The finest art* (2nd ed.). St. Louis, MO: Mosby–Yearbook, Inc.

Engebretson, J. (1998). A heterodox model of healing. *Alternative Therapies, 4* (2), 37–43.

Hall, L. E. (1963). A center for nursing. *Nursing Outlook, 11* (11), 805–806.

Hall, L. E. (1969). The Loeb Center for Nursing and Rehabilitation. *International Journal of Nursing Studies, 6,* 81–95.

Hensley, S. (1998). A world of difference. *Modern Healthcare, 28* (44), 24–28.

Loose, V. (1994). Lydia E. Hall: Rehabilitation nursing pioneer in the ANA hall of fame. *Rehabilitation Nursing, 19* (3), 174–176.

May, R. (1994). *The courage to create.* New York: W.W.Norton.

Montgomery, C. (1996). The care-giving relationship: Paradoxical and transcendent aspects. *Alternative Therapies, 2* (2), 52–57.

O'Connor, B. B. (1995). *Healing traditions: Alternative medicine and the health professions.* Philadelphia: University of Pennsylvania Press.

Tonges, M. C., Rothstein, H., & Carter, H. K. M. B. (1998). Sources of satisfaction in hospital nursing practice. *Journal of Nursing Administration, 28* (5), 47–61.

PART THREE

Caring Modalities: Nursing and Complementary Therapies

FLORENCE NIGHTINGALE SAYS IN HER BOOK, *NOTES ON NURSING,* that the purpose of nursing is to "put the patient in the best condition possible for nature to work upon him" (1969, p. 110). She said this based upon a belief that disease is a "reparative process" and that nursing is more than the "administration of medication and application of poultices" (p. 2). Nightingale's historical book details the importance of attending to the patient's environment and diet. She says, "So deep rooted and universal is the conviction that to give medicine is to be doing something, or rather everything; to give air, warmth, cleanliness, etc., is to do nothing . . . the exact value of particular remedies and modes of treatment is by no means ascertained, while there is universal experience as to the extreme importance of careful nursing in determining the issue of the disease" (p. 3).

Has anything really changed? Nurses still question whether their role has been reduced to that of providing medication and charting. How often do we chart, or get recognized for changing the temperature of a room, turning down the lights, or making a patient more comfortable? How often do we communicate to each other, on a care plan or face to face, these seemingly insignificant details of what Nightingale established as fundamental patient care? Do we demonstrate caring by finding out what the patient needs to be in the best condition possible for "nature to work upon him"?

There are many nursing subspecialty areas that are beginning to place greater value on the total environment of the patient and exploring new ways of addressing comfort. For example, many neonatal intensive care units (NICU) have implemented a model called the Newborn Individualized Developmental Care and Assessment Program (NIDCAP). This program emphasizes the environmental sensitivities of the premature infant and the ways in which a caregiver can provide an environment for the baby that allows nature to "work upon him." In an NICU, many of the babies are indeed working with nature and a "higher power" as they grow and develop in order to finish the work that is usually performed in the mother's womb. Nurses create developmentally sensitive environments for the babies and have found that babies have better medical outcomes and often leave the hospital sooner (Als & Gilkerson, 1997).

We might ask how this type of nursing attention to the environment, comfort level, and "best condition possible" might benefit *all* patients. The ongoing concern among nurses must be to discover what the "best position possible" is for the patient so that he can be healed by nature. This entails using the integrative nursing practices of keen observation and perceiving the patient's individual, holistic needs for care, finding ways to help the patient achieve and maintain balance or homeostasis, and using biomedical and caring skills to help patients. Putting the patient in the "best condition possible for nature to work upon him" implies that the nurses must know something about the science and art of caring. We must know something about the healing powers of "nature" herself. "Natural" remedies that are often used in complementary therapies are also discussed in nursing literature. As with any nursing modality, the use of natural remedies must be learned.

Nurses must examine any modality to be used in practice and attempt to gain greater insight into the science behind it, as well as the art of using the modality for the care of the patient. As mentioned previously many ancient healing traditions, such as the Native American traditions, believe that the healing is not *in* the object of healing, technique, or modality, but is found in the spirit of the healer and the person seeking healing. Healing as a spiritual act takes place in the relationship of the beings involved and is often transferred through the *object* of healing. This object might be a touch, a medicine, a healing environment, or a kind word. Caring modalities are objects of healing. Complementary therapies, drugs, and surgeries are all objects of healing. These objects are not in and of themselves healing to patients. It is in the use of these objects in creating evolving, healing relationships, and in demonstrating care that they become valuable to the health care experience of patients. As depicted in the healing relationship model below, nurses create "bonds" and "points of connection" as they interact with patients and make use of various objects of healing or modalities.

Parts One and Two of this book discussed the concepts of demonstrating care and integrative nursing as well as the ways nurses, both past and present, have demonstrated caring through their use of various techniques and modalities. The purpose of Part Three is to provide a closer examination of the five categories of modalities that have been part of the fundamentals of nursing care for decades and which are, at present, often referred to as "complementary therapies."

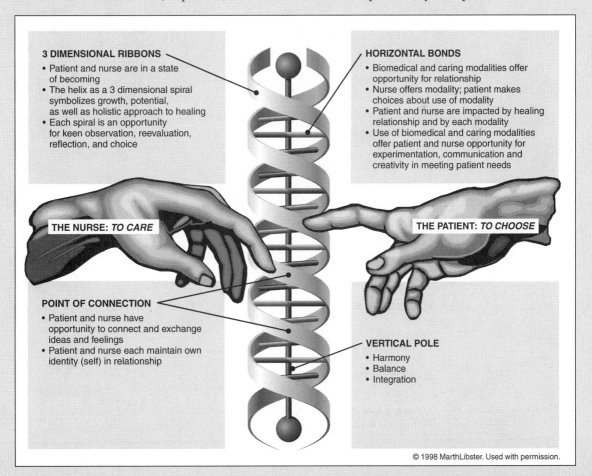

3 DIMENSIONAL RIBBONS
- Patient and nurse are in a state of becoming
- The helix as a 3 dimensional spiral symbolizes growth, potential, as well as holistic approach to healing
- Each spiral is an opportunity for keen observation, reevaluation, reflection, and choice

HORIZONTAL BONDS
- Biomedical and caring modalities offer opportunity for relationship
- Nurse offers modality; patient makes choices about use of modality
- Patient and nurse are impacted by healing relationship and by each modality
- Use of biomedical and caring modalities offer patient and nurse opportunity for experimentation, communication and creativity in meeting patient needs

THE NURSE: *TO CARE*

THE PATIENT: *TO CHOOSE*

POINT OF CONNECTION
- Patient and nurse have opportunity to connect and exchange ideas and feelings
- Patient and nurse each maintain own identity (self) in relationship

VERTICAL POLE
- Harmony
- Balance
- Integration

Chapter 6 explores the *world* of complementary therapies as *objects of healing* in preparation for taking a closer look at the caring modalities discussed in Chapters 7–11. The five modalities addressed in Part Three have been chosen for their historical significance to nursing. They are touch therapies, use of the environment such as hydrotherapy and plant use, nutrition, communication, and energy therapy. Although a nurse in practice today might think that some of these therapies, such as the use of "energy" in providing patient care, is a "new age" concept used by complementary therapy practitioners, it is common to find these therapies described in detail, including various forms of energy therapies (e.g., ray therapy, heliotherapy, and electric shock), in many historical nursing texts. Historical nursing texts also reveal that nurses were considered experts in the use of these modalities.

Chapters 7–11 discuss the history of one of these modalities in nursing practice, the art and science of using the modality as a means of demonstrating care, and how today's nurse might integrate the modality into practice. Each chapter includes a reference to an appendix of resources for further learning about the particular modality.

Nursing is at yet another crossroads where many of the caring modalities used throughout history are being looked at by governing bodies, professional organizations, the public, and nurses themselves as something very separate from fundamental nursing practice. For example, whether a nurse can advise a patient about nutrition has emerged as an issue. Can only a registered dietician provide food and nutrition information? Can a nurse provide a massage or does she need to get special education and a license independent from her nursing license? Who will provide holistic, total patient care in a health care system that continually specializes and subspecializes and is suspicious of the care provided by a generalist practitioner such as a professional nurse?

Is it possible that the caring modalities used by nurses throughout history have become so mundane that they no longer spark much interest among some in the profession? Or has the magic and effectiveness of these caring modalities been kept hidden away for so long that they are beginning to fade from our memories as well as our practice? Mary Chiarella, Director of Professional Services at New South Wales College of Nursing in Australia wrote, "I thought about all the times I had massaged patients' backs and they had expressed their pleasure, about all the times I held people's hands, made up their faces, washed them with soaps and shampoos that smelt of flowers and herbs. We knew the magic we were creating, but we kept it secret behind those screens didn't we? It was what I have previously described as the privilege of intimacy, but we stepped out from behind those screens and briskly reported on the integrity of Mr. Jones' skin, the patency of his canula and the drainage from his catheter and if you hadn't been there, you would never have known" (1995, p. 24).

It is my hope that by sharing the history of some of these modalities, ways they are being used in health care as complementary therapies, as well as my personal experience integrating them into nursing practice, that the reader might experience renewed curiosity and wonder about what these modalities mean to patients as well as to the future of nursing practice. "Carefully, tactfully, so as not to destroy the magic, the blend of body and spirit care which is nursing at its best is coming to the fore. Some of the natural therapies which nurses used in the past are being used again, and their value is being explored and wondered about in nursing work" (Chiarella, 1995, p. 24).

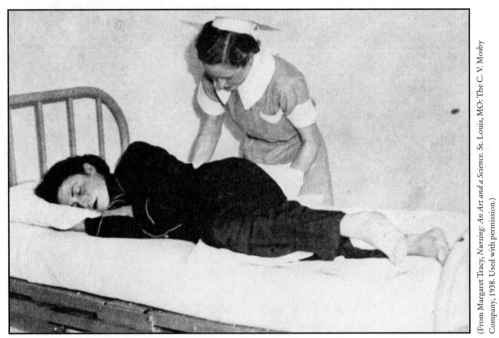

Positioning a patient, 1938

(From Margaret Tracy, *Nursing: An Art and a Science.* St. Louis, MO: The C. V. Mosby Company, 1938. Used with permission.)

The real voyage of discovery consists not in seeking new landscapes but in having new eyes.

—MARCEL PROUST

CHAPTER 6

A New Name for Nursing Fundamentals

Nursing Fundamentals

Florence Nightingale wrote about nursing fundamentals as specific tasks nurses perform to "put the patient in the best condition for nature to work upon him" (Nightingale, 1957, p. 75). She wrote about such duties as creating a healing environment, maintaining hygiene, and providing food. The basics or fundamentals of nursing care have never really changed throughout history. Years later, Virginia Henderson wrote a book, *Basic Principles of Nursing Care,* in which she defines basic nursing as addressing the "care that any person requires no matter what the physician's diagnosis and the therapy he prescribes although both influence the plan the nurse initiates and carries out. The nurse's basic care is the same whether the patient is considered physically or mentally ill" (1970, p. 1). She goes on to say that basic nursing can be applied in any setting and by nature is "preventative as well as curative" (p. 1). Many nurse theorists have focused on the role of the nurse as being one who helps the patient with basic human needs, activities of daily living, and interaction with society. Because nurses are often the only caregiver with twenty-four-hour responsibilities, they take on the most intimate of care, which is not addressed by other caregivers. The basic nursing tasks have been created to address the most fundamental human needs. The need for touch and interaction with the environment are as fundamental to human existence as are food and shelter. Nursing care and the modalities used in caring for others address these fundamental needs. Historical texts on nursing fundamentals include the patients' needs for breathing normally, eating and drinking, elimination, movement and positioning, sleep and rest, dress, body temperature, hygiene, environment, and communication. Nursing fundamentals address the sensory experience of the patient and their need for comfort.

COMFORT MEASURES

Comfort can be described as feeling *at ease.* Even when someone is *dis-eased,* it is possible for them to achieve a state in which they feel *at ease.* Comfort is achieved and experienced in different ways by different people. It is a subjective experience that is shaped by one's own cultural beliefs, habits, and memories. The manner in which a person comforts herself begins in infancy. In addition to finding out for themselves, babies learn from their parents what is and is not comforting. Some babies find thumb sucking to be comforting only to discover that their parents forbid the practice.

Providing comfort for someone is not as easy as it sounds. Nurses are expected to provide comfort as a way of demonstrating care. But what does a pediatric nurse do for a small child who desperately wants to suck his pacifier and the parents have said, "Don't let him suck his pacifier"? What does a nurse do for the patient who desperately needs to smoke a cigarette after surgery only to find that the hospital is a non-smoking hospital? Providing comfort is not as easy as it is often made out to be. There are many aspects of a comforting experience for someone. As discussed in nursing historical texts, sensory needs and cultural beliefs as well as fundamental human needs are all elements of the patient's unique, inherent knowledge of what it means to be comforted.

This knowledge is deeply stored in every cell of our being as *memory.* Remember the expression that "One man's medicine is another man's poison"? It is the same with comfort. What is comforting to one can be irritating or anxiety-provoking to another. Having always been intrigued by how people comfort themselves and others, I have often asked my patients what they think would be comforting for them in their time of need. I have had some very interesting responses that have shown me how much cultural beliefs, life-sensory experience, and memory influence the choices people make as to how they comfort and take care of themselves.

When I was a rural home care nurse, I visited a pregnant woman with hyperemesis. She had been vomiting for a number of days and was fast approaching the need for hospitalization. She had not called her doctor at first because she thought the vomiting would go away and she thought that she was able to care for herself. I talked with her and then started the IV fluids prescribed by her doctor. Then I asked her what would make her feel more comfortable, perhaps even able to hold down some food. Her answer is one I will never forget. She said, "I just know that I could hold down mashed potatoes." I thought to myself, "I can make that for her." Then she added, "With lettuce in it." I immediately had this image in my mind of a warm bowl of yummy mashed potatoes with green lettuce wilting in it, and swallowed hard. I told her I could make it for her right away. When I brought her the food, I asked her about the wilted lettuce. She said that her mother had given it to her when she was sick. Her mother is Dutch, and a potato with lettuce was something her own mother had given to family members who were ill. Needless to say, the patient kept down a whole bowl of potatoes with wilted lettuce. I have never had a patient since then who requested this particular food to control vomiting.

Potatoes and wilted lettuce was a comforting food for this patient. She got better with the IV fluids and the potato and lettuce. She felt better, too. The nursing goal was to help her maintain adequate hydration and hold down any food that she could. The patient and I accomplished this together. Demonstrating care is about providing comfort in a way that is familiar and nonthreatening to the patient. Patients often know what they need for comfort but they are either unable or unwilling to provide comfort for themselves. Nurses need to continue to explore the vast range of cultural differences and perceptions that exist in the *world* of caring modalities and comfort measures used by patients.

MEMORY AND SENSORY EXPERIENCE

People perceive their world through sensory experience. The five senses—taste, touch, smell, hearing, and seeing—enable us to know our environment and the people in that environment. Our senses also provide ways of developing relationships with our environment and other people. The fundamentals of nursing care address the sensory needs of patients, the need for relationship, and intimacy. This is why nursing fundamentals, or the basics in nursing, are intimate. But nursing fundamentals are more than basic; they are foundational to all other caregiving behaviors.

The senses provide information that the body, being such an adaptable organism, needs for survival. It needs continuous information about its environment in order to adapt or change to meet the need of the moment. This adaptation, also called homeostasis or balance, occurs on bodily and cellular levels. Sensory experiences are stored at cellular levels. "It is possible that the info-energy of any experience, including odor, sound and flavor, is stored on some level within all of the body's cells . . ." (Pearsall, 1998, p. 111). The sensory experience becomes memory. Cells have memory and are able to learn. For example, the cells of the immune system "remember" which substances entering the body are "invaders" and which are not. People not only learn cellularly, but they also learn viscerally and holistically (i.e., body, mind, and spirit) what things they engage in bring balance, homeostasis, and comfort. For example, many people learn what food upsets their stomach. They might also learn what food upsets their stomach only when they are emotionally upset.

Learning and experiencing what helps us stay in balance and *at ease* is healing. "On this oldest and most basic human sense level, an object transmits its info-energetic code, is turned into a cellular memory, and we not only sense our environment but

become it" (Pearsall, 1998, p. 112). Hence the importance of nurses' abilities to provide the "best condition possible for nature to work upon him" (the patient) so that
any adaptation and balance can occur. Hence the importance of using nursing fundamentals that provide the sensory experience, the environment, and the comfort necessary for healing.

Janice Morse writes, "Because of the acute care and curing orientation of the hospital, nursing comfort tasks are devalued and regarded by patients as non-technical,
ordinary, kind and helpful (but not essential or critical for cure). Thus this comfort
work becomes invisible, despite its therapeutic implications, and when nurses are
busy, comfort work receives a lower priority in the work schedule than medical or
mechanical tasks. This devaluation has become so pervasive that nurses themselves
do not consider their work to be comforting to patients. Indeed when Strauss et al.
(1984) identified five types of comfort work tasks that nurses assumed, these tasks
were identified in terms of dis-comfort: preparing patients for discomfort, preventing
discomfort . . ." (1992, p. 99).

If true, then perhaps nursing needs to reevaluate the importance of the nursing
modalities it calls "fundamentals" and how these daily tasks of providing nourishment, touch, a listening ear, a comfortable environment, energy, and light, often dele-

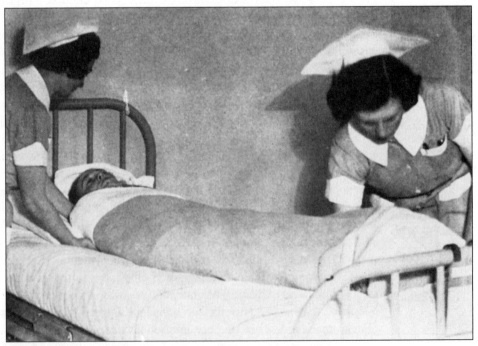

Nurse completing a full body wrap, 1938 *(From Margaret Tracy,* Nursing: An Art and a Science.
St. Louis, MO: The C.V. Mosby Company, 1938. Used with permission.)

gated to nursing assistants, are the heart of our service to life. Nurses need to assess whether or not their assistants are capable and willing to provide the comfort and sensory experience the patient needs and expects from a nursing service. Perhaps we need to explore further as well as reeducate the public about the importance of the fundamental caring modalities a patient can use in self-care or in the care of a family or friend. Nurses can look for creative ways to practice integrative nursing when providing professional patient care in which fundamental caring modalities are given equal value with biomedical tasks.

Total Healing Experience

Even though some members of society may, as Morse says, believe that comfort is not "critical or essential to cure," they certainly have not dismissed their need for comfort as part of their total health and healing experience. Many continue to seek comfort in their native cures. Many now turn to the complementary therapies (CT) or alternative medicine (AM) practitioner for health and healing needs once brought to the nurse or physician.

The Office of Alternative Medicine at the National Institutes of Health lists massage, diet, changes in lifestyle, and counseling as complementary and alternative medicine (CAM). At one time, science-based nursing was listed. This is because the working definition of CAM has been "any medical intervention not taught widely at U.S. medical schools or generally available at U.S. hospitals" (Eisenberg, 1993, p. 246). It is understandable that nursing would fit this definition. But from the viewpoint of being alternative to medicine? No. Is nursing complementary to medicine? Absolutely! Because nursing is "complementary" to medicine, and some of the historical caring practices of nursing are now being labeled by influential organizations as "complementary," I refer to these caring modalities as complementary rather than "alternative."

Another reason to refer to these practices as complementary is that research has shown that one in three people seeing a medical doctor also sees a CT practitioner (Eisenberg et al., 1998, p. 1572). Many Americans, Europeans, Australians, and Chinese, to name a few, seek their health care from many sources, within both the complementary and biomedical systems.

Nurses can gain a greater understanding of the modalities used in providing care by looking at the trends in health care choices made by members of a society. "Our nursing knowledge base will need to increasingly reflect the notion that health behaviors, illness experiences and nursing acts cannot be understood in isolation from the socio-cultural context that shapes their meaning" (Thorne, 1993, p. 1939). Nurses provide the care that a patient needs. As a profession, nurses advocate for patient rights and believe in assisting them in choices for self-care. But it is not an easy task when they work in a biomedical world that labels any health practice outside that which is taught in medical schools as "alternative." In discussing the apparent rift between biomedical and alternative medicine practitioners, Ellen Zagorsky states that, "Nursing seems to lie somewhere in the middle of these two approaches. Nurses must implement institutional policy when working with patients and families, but they also must be responsive to patients' beliefs, as well as patients' rights as consumers to influence the way their care is administered" (1993, p. 72). Nurses walk between two worlds.

What do consumers want? Complementary therapies to be sure. And they are willing to pay for them, too. In 1997, Americans made 629 million visits to CT practitioners and 58.3 percent of those paid for their visits out-of-pocket. This represents more visits than were made in 1997 to primary care physicians (Eisenberg et al., 1998, p. 1569). In 1997, Eisenberg reports that 42 percent of people who went to a CT practitioner did so to treat an existing illness. Fifty-eight percent went to "prevent future illness from occurring or to maintain health and vitality" (p. 1575). Is this so hard to believe when it was found in 1978 that, in general, "three quarters of physician-patient encounters are occasioned by complaints that are either self-limited, or for which medicine has no specific remedies. Such patients presumably benefit from seeing a doctor because he listens sympathetically to their words and then consoles and reassures them" (Ingelfinger, 1978, p. 945).

Yet research seems to show that patients are not leaving their biomedical practitioners. They continue to visit their biomedical practitioner as well as their CT practitioners. *Our patients are already using an integrative model for their health care!* It would be in keeping with our professional history to listen to the integrative needs and actions of our patients and make the appropriate changes in our practice to provide the comfort, support, and care for which we are known.

People turn to complementary therapies because "these health practices are more congruent with their own values, beliefs and philosophical orientations towards health and life" (Astin, 1998, p. 1548). There has been no significant correlation between race, gender, negative attitudes toward conventional medicine, or the desire for control over health practice and the use of CT. The Astin study showed that having a holistic philosophy of health was indeed predictive of CT use. Because nursing practice is based upon a holistic framework, it is not surprising that many nurses have been exploring the possibility of using CT in practice.

In one survey of 393 nurses, more than half had used CT in practice, in particular massage and aromatherapy. Eighty-eight percent of those using CT had undergone some formal training (Trevelyan, 1996, p. 42). This survey found that most nurses used the CT for purposes of relaxation, stress reduction, pain relief, insomnia, pregnancy, labor, and palliative care. "Less than one percent stated that the therapies had no effect on their patients. 88.5% said that they had definitely seen improvement" (p. 42).

Many years ago, before I entered the healing professions, I decided to look into healing practices I had heard about from friends. These practices were very different from the things I had learned from my doctors as I was growing up. My family often used self-care practices and usually only called the doctor for emergencies. We used salves and steam, castor oil, and Merthiolate. We had our own organic vegetable and herb garden and we tried to follow Grandpa's example of chewing our food thoroughly. He chewed every bite forty-seven times! My grandfather was also the one who used to give freshly squeezed aloe vera juice to his friends who had stomach ulcers. He used to tell them to drink the juice of the "burn plant" because "the ulcer is a burn." It always sounded like common sense to me and it worked, too. Because of my experience with my family's healing practices, it was not hard for me to understand that many people had their own way of healing themselves.

I received a baccalaureate degree in 1981 from New York University in dance therapy, a modality now included on the National Center for Complementary and Alternative Medicine (NCCAM) list. Back then, I learned that people did not always respond to the more common talking therapies. I worked with autistic children and found that movement was a much better therapy to use when trying to enter their world. I found it to be true in nursing, too, that not all people respond to the same therapy. One person's medicine is another person's poison. I found that having a repertoire, or a series of caring modalities to choose from, made it easier for me when interacting with patients. I found that a modality was often the key to opening the door of the patient's heart, as well as my own, and that the caring modality was often the catalyst for the healing relationship to begin.

The fact that complementary therapies "work" in providing healing and comfort, and that they are often the familiar health care choice, are only two of the reasons for nurses to examine the use of CT in practice. Cost is also an important factor. Cost to the patient is not only measured financially. It is also measured by its impact upon health and longevity. Complementary therapies are often significantly cheaper than the drugs, surgeries, and tests that are so common in the biomedical world. Dr. Alan Gaby prepared a report for the NCCAM on the cost effectiveness of certain CAM practices. For example, the treatment of benign prostatic hyperplasia with surgery and pharmaceutical drugs for one patient was stated to be $5,540. An effective medical treatment with a standardized herbal extract of saw palmetto berries was $150 per person annually (Gaby, personal communication, April 10, 1999).

Many pharmaceutical drugs and practices, although potentially life saving, can also have significant side effects. Many CTs do not have the same risk of side effects as the more invasive treatments. However, no assumptions of safety can be made about any modality used in nursing practice. Safety and research are very important issues regardless of the modality. "As health providers, we can participate in alternative/complementary therapies on many levels, from merely assessing what therapies a patient has tried, to helping patients evaluate and identify suitable complementary therapy providers, to becoming trained in complementary therapy, to doing research on the effectiveness of complementary therapies. All of these levels of participation

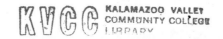

in complementary therapies presuppose that we are continuously learning about them and the more traditional therapies we may more routinely apply" (Tiedje, 1998, p. 561). Regardless of our level of involvement in complementary therapies, and because of the similarity of complementary therapies and nursing fundamentals, nurses *will* be involved in some way with the expansion and integration of complementary therapies and health care. It is yet to be seen how nursing as a profession will establish its position on this subject. Nurses must seriously consider the history of these caring modalities and the need for continuing the work of those who went before us by researching and enhancing the modalities that have been used in practice throughout the history of our profession.

The Challenge of Research in Complementary Therapies

There are three things nurses often say to me when I talk with them about developing caring modalities (i.e., complementary therapies) in nursing practice. "What about supporting research? Aren't a lot of those therapies placebos? What about the safety issues in using these therapies?" These are important questions. Researching complementary therapies used in nursing practice is challenging for the same reason that research on caring or research in other disciplines, such as psychiatry, is challenging. The art and science of healing involves many variables that cannot always be controlled.

Dr. J. William LaValley writes that, "Standardization, randomization, isolation and control are difficult to apply to research on complementary health care because reductionist isolation of each variable destroys the holistic, non-linear approach involved in complementary health care and fails to account for the unique aspects of each patient" (LaValley & Verhoef, 1995, p. 48). As David Lukoff, PhD, points out in his article on researching complementary therapies, many patients who use complementary therapies use more than one treatment modality, which challenges our ability to understand any research outcomes. Nursing also involves the use of more than one modality. He says, "The highly regarded randomized controlled clinical trial, though often powerful and useful, is neither feasible nor ideal for understanding the effects of many unconventional treatment approaches" (Lukoff, Edwards, & Miller, 1998, p. 44). Even medicine is not immune to these research concerns. Robert Gatchel writes that, "There is increasing need in medicine for appropriately conducted outcome research, especially randomized controlled trials leading to inferences about causality. Many 'established' medical fields still lack substantial and high-quality treatment-outcome research. This shortcoming is therefore not limited to alternative therapies" (Gatchel & Maddrey, 1998, p. 36). The United States Office of Technology Assessment did a study that suggested that only 20 percent of modern medical remedies in common use have been scientifically proved to be effective (Brown, 1998).

Nurses often have firsthand experience as to the evidence of this statement. As a nurse caring for children, I witnessed physicians continuously prescribe medications never tested on children. I also witnessed physicians prescribe cardiovascular health regimes for women that had only been tested on men. And I have witnessed physicians and their mentally ill, pregnant patients agonize over prescribing a psychiatric drug for the mother, knowing that the risk to the fetus is all but unknown. Nurses know how difficult it is to find research that offers greater understanding when decisions such as these must be made.

The same issues are found in nursing practice. We have a tremendous need for published clinical research that can illuminate the holistic nature of our practice, as well as provide justification for the time and expense of providing certain modalities to patients. Randomized clinical trials might be the gold standard approach for drug testing but they are often inadequate in providing insight into the health beliefs, nurse-patient relationships, and caring modalities that are part of the scope of nursing practice.

There are alternatives, however, to quantitative research designs such as randomized clinical trials that can be used to study complementary therapies and nurses' caring modalities. One example is case study design. Case studies provide an in-depth exploration of a single patient's health experience. They provide a model and a means for "transforming the 'anecdotal' into a disciplined inquiry of individual cases. As a research tool, the case study method can provide descriptive, exploratory data—both qualitative and quantitative—from multiple sources that are sensitive to the contemporary context within which the experience takes place" (Lukoff et al., 1998, p. 44). The case study method requires keen observation, a quality Florence Nightingale herself valued. Those who have become enamored of quantitative designs often dismiss case studies as prescientific or preexperimental. ". . . Case studies are the preferred strategy when 'how' and 'why' questions are being posed, when the investigator has little control over events, and when the focus is on a contemporary phenomenon within some real-life context. Case studies have played an important role in documenting the existence of rare disorders in which the researcher cannot control the phenomenon or even identify a large subject pool" (Lukoff et al., 1998, p. 45). Another important argument for the use of case study methodology by nurses is that it allows the nurse to integrate formal research methods into her everyday work. The caring work that nurses perform daily is often worth studying, discussing, and publishing as research.

There are numerous ways of investigating the therapeutic effects of caring modalities and complementary therapies. The Quantitative Methods Working Group convened by the NCCAM alone was able to identify numerous methodologies applicable to complementary therapies research (Dossey, 1998). In nursing we have many qualitative designs to choose from as well. Often a combined approach of quantitative and qualitative design is most appropriate.

What does all this talk of research mean to patient care? Do patients really care whether or not a therapy has been studied? In the case of fundamental care they often do not. Many of the choices people make regarding the complementary therapies they use are based upon their vernacular health beliefs. For example, if I were to develop a stomach ulcer, I might just drink aloe juice because I saw my grandfather help many people heal their ulcers with it. Firsthand knowledge and experience is very valuable when making health decisions. Dr. Bonnie O'Connor writes, "While many members of the general populace also esteem and seek scientific information, they do not invariably feel it is the only—or even the best—way to acquire or confirm certain kinds of knowledge. They do not necessarily believe it to be free from bias and corruption, or find its pronouncements trustworthy solely on the basis of their source. Nor do they regard it as the final arbiter of the truth" (O'Connor, 1995, p. 15).

Nurses know that patients may have no interest in the supporting research for the modality they choose to use in comforting themselves or their loved one. As we approach the question of the importance of research in caring modalities, it is best to remember that research and scientific knowledge are part of our Western health care culture, part of our worldview, but not necessarily part of the worldview or culture of the patients we serve. In integrating biomedical and caring skills, we must approach research from the standpoint of being one "piece of the clinical puzzle" and certainly not the "whole picture." Many things influence our choice of caring modalities; most importantly our relationship with the individual patient. The purpose of researching caring modalities is to provide insight as to how to better "put the patient in the best condition for nature to work upon him." Our scientific research and observations are not nature itself, but rather nature exposed to our method of questioning.

THE SCIENCE AND MAGIC OF PLACEBO

Some nurses tend to dismiss the positive effects they observe when providing care to patients as being due to placebo, as if there were something wrong with a placebo effect. Placebo effect itself has been scientifically studied for depressed patients, for example, and found to have a success rate of 30 percent to 40 percent (Brown, 1998, p. 91). In another study, it was found that "70% of cases of angina pectoris respond well to placebo" (Luskin et al., 1998, p. 47). The use of placebo is one of the oldest forms of healing.

A placebo is defined as any treatment or aspect of treatment that does not have a specific action on the patient's symptoms or disease. Placebo, which in Latin means, "I shall please," has formed the primary basis of medical care until approximately one hundred fifty years ago when antibiotics were discovered (Luskin et al., 1998). The placebo effect is not completely understood, but it is thought that a placebo provides reassurance, decreases fear or anxiety, and provides hope to patients. "Placebos seem to be most reliably effective for afflictions in which stress directly affects the symptoms such as pain, high blood pressure, depression and asthma (Brown, 1998, p. 93). In short, placebos provide comfort.

Patients who are told by a health practitioner that they will feel better often experience the reassurance they need. They often get better. Is this a placebo effect? Patients in a study at State University of New York Downstate Medical Center in Brooklyn who were told that they would be inhaling an allergen through a nebulizer, when it was only saline, developed problems with airway obstruction. When they were given another nebulizer treatment, and told that it was medicine that would help, their airways opened up again (Brown, 1998, p. 93). The power of placebo and suggestion in the hands of a trusted health practitioner cannot be underestimated.

Nurses often underestimate the healing power of the trusted relationship *they* have with patients. A nurse's very presence has the potential of being highly influential in the outcome of care to the patient. Nurses often provide the reassurance the patient needs to heal as they go about the care of the patient. "Physicians and nurses of yesterday seemed to understand the importance of a good bedside manner. Many of today's medical experts still appreciate the healing power of a compassionate consultation, but under pressure to provide "cost-effective" care, they (and particularly insurance companies) may be losing sight of this crucial component of effective care" (Brown, 1998, p. 94).

What nurses do may seem like magic or placebo. As of yet it is not completely apparent what the role of nursing presence and caring modalities, like placebo, will be in the future of health care. But until the investigation has truly begun, is there any harm in providing caring modalities that seem to be effective? Is there any harm in providing caring modalities that the public continues to seek out in their journey to find a little bit of comfort?

Safety Issues

The risks and benefits of any caring modality or complementary therapy for a particular patient must be discussed when helping a patient decide whether or not a modality is appropriate for him. It is really no different than checking a heart rate before giving digoxin. Just because a massage is often beneficial for bedridden patients does not mean that *every* bedridden patient will benefit from a massage. For example, many physically healthy pregnant women who are required to be bedridden for any period of time during their pregnancy might find a massage soothing and helpful to their circulation. But if the woman became pregnant as the result of rape, and experienced tremendous fear and pain every time she was touched, she might not want a massage. A massage might be contraindicated for her at least until that point in her therapy when touch can be therapeutic, rather than traumatic. Nurses who use complementary therapies must be sensitive and observant of the appropriate use of any modality. A nursing text from 1938 states that "Mastery of the simple mechanics of nursing procedures is easily gained. Unless that mastery is coupled with an appreciation of how and when they should be used, when and in what ways they should be modified, what reactions can be expected from the patient and for what danger signals the nurse should be alert, it is dangerous. A proper discipline is conscientious acting on intelligent understanding" (Tracy, 1938, p. 30).

Caring modalities are tailored to the individual needs of patients. It is best to use modalities that are in keeping with a patient's belief system and expectations. It is important to assess health and cultural beliefs prior to suggesting any caring modality; otherwise establishing a healing relationship may become a challenge. I once saw a patient with a diagnosed conversion disorder, a condition in which she was unable to walk, but there was no discoverable physiologic reason for her not to walk. A practitioner suggested to her that she have hypnosis before interviewing her to find out more about her health beliefs. The client became very defensive at the suggestion of hypnosis and told me later that her family was Baptist and was opposed to hypnosis. She subsequently rejected any further care from the other practitioner. The practitioner could have improved the healing relationship with the patient by including a spirituality assessment prior to proposing hypnosis. The practitioner could also have explored the social understanding and controversies about hypnosis as a modality prior to offering it to the patient.

In addition to appropriateness related to patient belief and readiness for a therapy, the safe use of caring modalities or complementary therapies also implies being aware of the interaction of all the therapies a patient is using. Subtle interactions can occur between two or more noninvasive therapies and between noninvasive therapies and invasive therapies. A nurse might observe the patient who uses two noninvasive therapies such as guided imagery and massage. Or a nurse might work with a patient who is taking herbal medicine and getting chiropractic treatments. The greatest area of concern is when patients are using multiple invasive therapies, such as taking two different drugs or combining a drug with an herbal supplement.

Nurses using fundamental caring modalities in practice today, such as touch therapies, nutrition, communication, energy therapies, and creating a healing environment, need to know as much about their patient as possible before implementing a plan of care that includes these modalities. Because many people are already using multiple modalities in self-care, as well as biomedical care, nurses are at greater risk of creating confusion, anxiety, and detrimental modality interactions when introducing another modality.

Much of the work in these five areas of fundamental caring modalities is subtle and, as said before, often goes unnoticed. An example might be turning off the lights in a room when a patient has dozed off for a nap. However, nurses are also becoming active in developing and researching some of these modalities to be used in a more direct therapeutic way. Nurses are researching massage, aromatherapy, reflexology, and therapeutic touch, to name a few. There is a big difference between holding a hand and providing a therapeutic touch healing treatment for a patient. Safety becomes more important as these caring modalities are developed in practice.

Continuing education is needed to address the ongoing safety issues in the use of complementary therapies and caring modalities. The final chapters of Part Three provide an introduction to complementary therapies and fundamentals in nursing care.

Conclusion

Chapters 7–11 discuss what are historically the five general headings of caring fundamentals. These five headings are touch, environment, nutrition, communication, and energy. A book could probably be written about each modality and its importance to nursing. Instead, a brief overview is given as an introduction to the modality. For those who have studied a particular modality in detail, the information given here may seem somewhat limited. I apologize in advance. It is my intention to provide insight into the healing experience that nurses provide patients through these modalities, the history behind the modality, and ways that nurses can continue to integrate these modalities into practice. If you find even one modality that is to your liking, and you see some opportunity for developing and integrating it into your caring practice, it will be enough.

I remind you of two things as you read Chapters 7–11. One is that, although some research has been included here, there is still a tremendous opportunity for more research in all five areas of caring practice. Two, as you consider what modalities you may want to integrate into your practice, keep in mind that more is not necessarily better; simplicity is often best.

References

Astin, J. (1998). Why patients use alternative medicine. *Journal of the American Medical Association, 279* (19), 1548–1553.

Brown, W. A. (1998). The placebo effect. *Scientific American, 278* (1), 90–95.

Chiarella, M. (1995). The magic of nursing. *Australian Nursing Journal, 3* (3), 22–24.

Dossey, L. (1998). The right man syndrome: Skepticism and alternative medicine. *Alternative Medicine, 4* (3), 12–19, 108–114.

Eisenberg, D. (1993). Unconventional medicine in the United States. *New England Journal of Medicine, 328* (4), 246–252.

Eisenberg, D., Davis, R., Ettner, S., Appel, S., Wilkey, S., Van Rompay, M., & Kessler, R. (1998). Trends in alternative medicine use in the United States, 1990–1997. *Journal of the American Medical Association, 280* (18), 1569–1575.

Gatchel, R., & Maddrey, A. M. (1998). Clinical outcome research in complementary and alternative medicine: An overview of experimental design and analysis. *Alternative Therapies, 4* (5), 36–42.

Henderson, V. (1970). *Basic principles of nursing care* (6th ed.). Geneva, Switzerland: International Council of Nurses.

Ingelfinger, F. (1978). Medicine: Meritorious or meretricious. *Science, 200,* 942–946.

LaValley, J. W., & Verhoef, M. (1995). Integrating complementary medicine and health care services into practice. *Canadian Medical Association Journal, 153* (1), 45–49.

Lukoff, D., Edwards, D., & Miller, M. (1998). The case study as a scientific method for researching alternative therapies. *Alternative Therapies, 4* (2), 44–52.

Luskin, F., Newell, K., Griffith, M., Holmes, M., Telles, S., Marvasti, F., Pelletier, K., & Haskell, W. (1998). A review of the mind-body therapies in the treatment of cardiovascular disease. *Alternative Therapies, 4* (3), 46–61.

Morse, J. (1992). Comfort. *Clinical Nursing Research, 1* (1), 91–106.

Nightingale, F. (1957). *Notes on nursing.* Philadelphia: J. B. Lippincott Co.

Nightingale, F. (1969). *Notes on nursing.* New York: Dover.

O'Connor, B. B. (1995). *Healing traditions: Alternative medicine and the health professions.* Philadelphia: University of Pennsylvania Press.

Pearsall, P. (1998). *The heart's code.* New York: Broadway Books.

Thorne, S. (1993). Health belief systems in perspective. *Journal of Advanced Nursing, 18,* 1931–1941.

Tiedje, L. B. (1998). Alternative health care: An overview. *Journal of Obstetrics, Gynecology, and Neonatal Nursing, 27,* 557–562.

Tracy, M. (1938). *Nursing: An art and a science.* St. Louis, MO: C.V. Mosby Co.

Trevelyan, J. (1996). A true complement? *Nursing Times, 92* (5), 42–43.

Zagorsky, E. (1993). Caring for families who follow alternative health care practices. *Pediatric Nursing, 19* (1), 71–74.

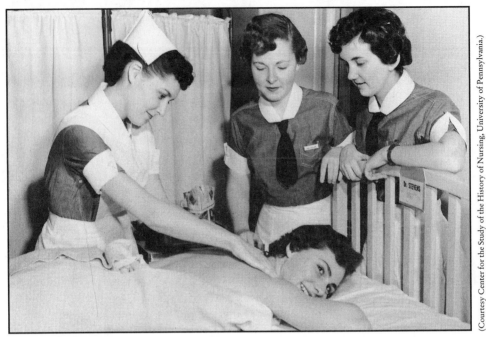

Effleurage

*The best and most beautiful things in the world cannot be
seen or even touched. They must be felt with the heart.*

—HELEN KELLER

CHAPTER 7

Touch: Opening the Door to the Heart

The History of Touch in Nursing Practice

Understanding the history of a caring modality is vital to understanding its development as a part of the art and a science of nursing practice. The historical use of touch is recorded at least as far back as the time of Hippocrates, the "father" of modern medicine, who is credited with saying that the key to health is to have an aromatic bath and a scented massage every day (Lawless, 1998). Throughout the history of nursing, massage and its simpler form, touch, have been part of the care provided to patients. Nursing is considered a "hands-on" profession. "The element of touch has proved to be extremely significant in nursing care. When no other method or technique is available, when nothing more can be done, human touch is always available to soothe, comfort, and to convey caring, compassion, and love" (Donahue, 1996, p. 22). Most nurses would agree that touch is integral to nursing practice.

Historical literature about nursing practice does not include the concept of touch per se. There are many references to nursing *tasks* that involve touching the patient. All bedside care such as bathing, positioning, and back rubs, involved purposeful touch on the part of the nurse. The importance of touch itself to nursing practice has only been written about in nursing literature in the past few decades.

Carole Estabrooks, a nurse who has researched the historical use of touch in nursing practice, writes that "the lack of extensive literature on how to touch is due to 'inherently' possessed prescriptive rules of the art of nursing. . . . Perhaps nurses wrote about touch implicitly because it was so much a part of seeming common sense and everyday practice that it did not seem necessary to describe touch explicitly" (1987, p. 42). Massage, rubbing, and effleurage have all been part of the daily care of patients for centuries.

Historically, there have been three reasons nurses touch patients. Nurses touch to comfort, to perform a procedure, or to do both. Some examples of procedural touch are bathing, percussion and postural drainage, and massage for therapeutic reasons such as stimulating circulation. Comforting touch is often used by nurses for relaxing a patient, promoting sleep, and for reassurance when the patient is upset. Nurses often use touch for both procedural and comfort reasons, such as when they are trying to minimize the discomfort caused by a particular task.

I have used touch for both reasons when giving immunizations to small children. I teach parents to use touch prior to the injection to warm the area and to increase the blood supply to the area that will be injected. Medications that are injected are often irritating and the child is better off if the medicine is absorbed quickly. I use touch to help the child relax her muscles so that the needle will penetrate the muscle more easily. Then I use touch after the injection for comfort, to "plug up the hole," and to reassure the child. I have found that shots are better tolerated with the integration of touch as part of the intervention.

In the 1970s, touch began to be recognized more for its contribution to nonverbal communication. Nurses have used touch as a way of saying, "I care. I am here to support you." Touch "conveys powerful messages of comfort, care and control to patients" according to a study called "Patients' Perceptions of Nurses' Use of Touch" (Mulaik et al., 1991, p. 319). This study showed that patients often have some ambivalence toward being touched by nurses. Sometimes nurses touch in ways that are not comforting, such as when doing wound care or helping a postoperative patient get out of bed for the first time. Indirectly or directly, the touch of the nurse can sometimes be associated in the mind of the patient with pain or discomfort.

In the narrative accounts in Chapter 4, all of the nurses identified touch, such as massage, effleurage, and handholding, as a way to demonstrate care that they had used throughout their careers. The difference between the use of touch by the retired nurses and the nurses in practice was that the retired nurses used rubbing and massage as a standard part of caring protocol. The nurses practicing today viewed massage as something they did as an "enhancement" to care or as something they do if they have the time. Mower writes of the return of massage to nursing practice, "When there was relatively little technology, it was part of the established protocol for nurses to rub down patients in their care" (Mower, 1997, p. 47). Patients do not expect a massage anymore when they come to a hospital. I have had patients act completely surprised when I offered a massage. During her narrative, Mary, a retired nurse, spoke about her own experience of being hospitalized and not receiving bedtime care that included a back rub as "they used to do for patients." This is not really surprising because nursing education often does not specifically include the art and science of

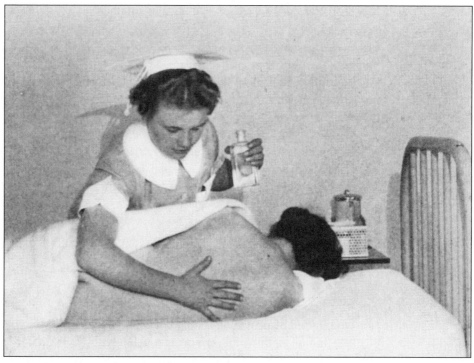

Back rub with warm oil, 1938 *(From Margaret Tracy,* Nursing: an Art and a Science. *St. Louis, MO: The C.V. Mosby Company, 1938. Used with permission.)*

touch. (Nurse massage therapists interviewed by Mower said that they received training in massage at massage therapy schools after their nursing education.) "Nursing education simply provided them limited knowledge of gentle strokes conducive to relaxation" (1997, p. 50). Perhaps the *basic* science and art of touch and touch therapies should be covered in a basic nursing curriculum as well as providing electives in touch therapies for nurses who wish to develop their skills of touch. "If touch has always been the special mark of the nursing profession—its way of making its unique and special presence felt by those in need of comfort and care, then it is important that it be understood" (Estabrooks, 1987, p. 46).

The Art and Science of Demonstrating Care through Touch

One of the most comprehensive books on the subject of the significance of touch is a book by Ashley Montagu called *Touching,* in which the author discusses the physiological effects of touching. Touch involves three major biological systems of the human body: the nervous system, the integument system, and the immune system. Although the connection between the sense of touch and the nervous and integument systems is well known, the concept of touch, i.e., skin-to-skin contact, having an immunologic function has been studied only recently. "The skin it has been found, more particularly its most superficial layer, the epidermis, produces a substance immunochemically indistinguishable from thymopoietin, the hormone of the thymus gland active in producing T-cell differentiation. T-cells are responsible for cellular immunity" (Montagu, 1986, p. 198). Animal studies have shown that maternal separation, loss of skin-to-skin contact, can suppress immune function in babies. Evidence has also been found that "there are significant biochemical differences between humans who have enjoyed adequate tactile stimulation and those who have not" (p. 201). It is well known that children who are not touched and cared for are at risk for developmental delays and significant health problems. Is it hard to believe that touch would be an important need for all humans regardless of age, sex, education, or social status? Montagu compares the physiologic effects of touch deprivation to that of maternal deprivation. He says that in both cases the physiological effects can be described by the word "shock." He also says that just as the treatment for shock is to replace the lost fluids, give oxygen and glucose, etc., so the shock of touch deprivation is remedied by providing touch. Touch is a powerful healing modality.

The immune-stimulating effects of touch can also be experienced indirectly. One study published in *Psychology and Health* with 132 college students was developed to study the effects of positive emotions on salivary IgA levels (one measure of immune response). In order to produce emotion in the students, half watched a documentary movie about the power struggles in World War II and half watched a documentary about Mother Theresa using touch to minister to the poor and sick in Calcutta, India. The movie about Mother Theresa was seen as inspiring and produced positive emotions in the audience. The study found that this group had significantly increased salivary IgA concentrations, indicating a heightened immune response (McClelland & Kirshnit, 1988). Perhaps this study is just the beginning of research to show that the demonstration of caring through touch by the Mother Theresas of this world, including nurses, has a profound effect on the immune systems of an entire community, whether or not they are the direct recipients of care.

Human touch deprivation not only manifests in physical symptoms, but is also exhibited as emotions such as loneliness, frustration, depression, and a lack of emotional warmth. When I worked in nursing homes I often found my elderly patients reaching out for a hug or a simple touch. They were genuinely isolated even though they were in homes with many other humans. Although the back rubs nurses provide to these patients might seem to "just make them feel good," it is a caring act of which the importance must not be taken lightly. Touch is critical to all patients' well-being and health.

Touch is an aspect of human experience that helps people know where they are in space and what their boundaries are. By touching the skin, people get to know where they end and the environment they live in begins. The importance of this type of "boundary knowing" might be better understood by comparing it to the experience of floating alone in the ocean. It quickly becomes uncomfortable for someone floating in the middle of an ocean to not be able to feel the bottom of the ocean with his toes or even to see the land occasionally. The drifting person begins to seek out something to hold on to as a way to relieve anxiety. A person who is blind does the same thing in an unfamiliar room. They begin by exploring the boundaries of the room defined by the walls, furniture, and other objects.

It is really no different for any human being, from the newborn whose place in space is no longer defined by the womb, to the elderly patient sitting in a chair all day without human contact. Whether or not patients demonstrate it physically, they are "reaching out" in some way and sometimes touch is the most expedient, reassuring way of letting them know where they are in space, that they are connected, and that someone cares. Often social norms and differences in culture keep people from reaching out for, or accepting, touch from nurses. Nurses need to assess the patient's ability to receive touch as well as his response to touch—whether touch is done as part of a procedure, for comfort, or both.

Part of the assessment of a patient's comfort level implies assessing the patient's ability to cope with pain. The effects of touch, most specifically massage, on pain have been studied. One study, by Weinrich and Weinrich, regarding pain management in cancer patients was based upon the gate control theory of pain and the idea that techniques such as massage close the gate to the central nervous system so that the patient *perceives* and experiences a decrease in pain. The study found that massage was helpful for males, but not females, and was of greater help to those subjects in the study who were experiencing high levels of pain. "The pilot study provides support for the use of alternative methods of pain alleviation such as massage in males, simultaneously with medication" (1990, p. 144).

Touch has also been used for pain management with women in labor. Nurses have often used massage to relieve the pain felt by the mother during a contraction. Massage therapists are trained to identify which massage techniques are appropriate within each stage and context of the laboring process. There is an art to choosing the appropriate touch technique for a particular patient and/or a particular condition.

The art of touch can be defined as the *way* in which a nurse demonstrates contact with a patient through touch. How a nurse demonstrates caring through touch has a lot to do with the purpose of the use of touch. As discussed before, nurses use touch during procedures and when comforting a patient. Routasalo and Lauri define a third category of touch as that of "therapeutic touching." They say that, "In therapeutic touching, the hands are used to lead human energy into the sick individual for the purpose of healing" (1996, p. 293). The hands are capable of being energy conduits, so to speak, for the nurse to use when assisting the movement of the patient's *own* energy.

All these uses of touch can be learned by the nurse. Routasalo writes that, "Estabrooks and Morse, using the method of grounded theory, observed that the nurse's touching style is learned; their cultural background and professional training as well as their experience with patients and the feedback they receive from them, all affect the learning process . . . touching situations are always different because the use of non-necessary touching depends on the nurse, the patient and daily variables" (1996, p. 295, 298).

Touch is truly an art and a caring skill used to comfort patients. The nurse needs to have a full understanding of the impact touch has upon patients physiologically, emotionally, and spiritually. Nurses must demonstrate care through touch by being judicious and respectful in how touch is used in practice. Being respectful when touching means recognizing the patient's boundaries, and the right to choose whether to be touched. There are many patient populations who, due to age or condition, cannot give consent to be touched. Infants, children, the elderly, and the comatose are examples. In cases of procedural or comforting touch, "telling" patients, either verbally or nonverbally, that they are about to be touched demonstrates respect. "Telling" nonverbally might mean slowly touching an extremity and watching for a response. Sometimes using both nonverbal and verbal "telling" is appropriate. If the touch being considered is for therapeutic reasons, the patient or guardian must give consent.

In my work with many types of health practitioners, I have noticed that those who touch patients a lot sometimes forget to respect patients' boundaries, their body. When we touch, we are performing a very intimate act and it is our responsibility to our patients to demonstrate our respect for the intimacy of the touch.

Often we know best how to respect others by how we have been respected. I once went to a chiropractor for a painful condition for which I received a physical spinal manipulation. After the chiropractor did the adjustment he left his hands on my spine to provide warmth and reassurance to the area of my back that had just experienced a tremendous jolt. I felt wonderful afterwards and was pain free. In contrast, I once worked in a clinic with a chiropractor who would often see patients in passing outside the office, talk with them about their complaint, and before the person knew it, the chiropractor would have reached up and "adjusted" their neck. There was no consent, no preparation, and no respect. This kind of touch can be traumatizing to patients. Learning when and what kind of touch is uncomfortable for patients is part of the keen observation practiced by integrative nurses.

Regardless of the research and experience around a particular touch modality, it is the responsibility of the nurse who uses that modality to assess its appropriateness for the holistic care of the patient at that moment. The quality of the practitioner's touch is an important part of the development of the patient-therapist relationship. Montagu writes about the importance of the work of movement analysts Bartenieff and Lewis, who note that, "Touch can vary in shape and effort, such as the elements from a fleeting light poke or a sudden poke, to a constricting two-dimensional grip, to a supportive, reassuring and sustained, slightly bound hold or to an indirect enveloping hold. Touch should be a form of three-dimensional shaping, they suggest, which is supportive rather than a form of more linear impositions such as poking" (Montagu, 1986, pp. 281–282).

Although, as nurses, we are often forced to do the poking type of touch to save a life, we must never forget our role to "shape" a touch for the patient so that is it comforting and reassuring.

Touch and Integrative Nursing

Nursing is a hands-on profession. Most nurses understand the value of touch in doing procedures and providing comfort to patients. They continue to strive for patient assignments and staffing levels that allow time for nurses to attend to the touch needs of patients. Nurses are not always familiar with the *therapeutic* uses of touch being developed by other nurses and by complementary therapy practitioners. The following are some examples, by no means exhaustive, of the types of touch modalities that may be useful in integrated nursing care.

FOOT REFLEXOLOGY

Much of my professional training in the art of touch was learned from a German therapist named Oma, which means grandmother. I apprenticed in Oma's foot reflexology clinic in California for two years while I attended nursing school. Foot reflexology is a type of foot massage that dates back at least to 2330 BC, 6th dynasty, Egypt. Footwork has been practiced for centuries throughout Europe and Asia. It is the practice of using specific hand and finger techniques to stimulate the reflexes in the feet that correspond to body tissues, organs, glands, and energy centers. It is not considered a medical treatment nor is it just a foot rub.

Foot reflexology work is based upon a number of theories. One is the holographic theory, that every body part contains the blueprint of the whole body. The foot is a hologram of the entire body, a scaled down version of the entirety (see Figure 7–1). Stimulating the foot sends a signal to the brain, a holographic organ, which has a connection to the blueprint of wholeness for that individual.

The late Dr. William Fitzgerald, an American physician who used reflexology/zone therapy techniques during the early part of the century, describes another theory of how reflexology works (Fitzgerald & Bowers, 1917). He said that the body is divided into ten zones and that the pressure applied to the areas of the foot in a particular zone affects any organ that lies in the corresponding zone in the body. Another theory is that the nerve endings in the foot are blocked by uric acid crystals which then block the flow of energy through the foot and therefore to the whole body. American reflexologists, Barbara and Kevin Kunz, of the Reflexology Research Center in Albuquerque, New Mexico, theorize that the effects of reflexology have to do

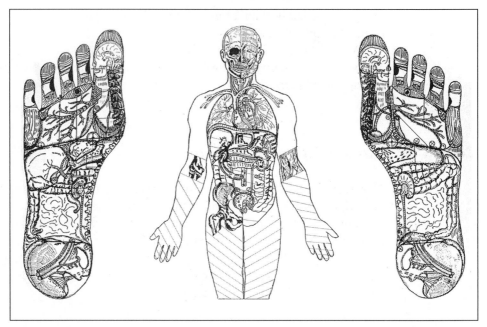

FIGURE 7-1
Example of a foot reflexology chart *(Courtesy Charles Ersdal and Christine Horvath. Used with permission.)*

with the stimulation of proprioceptive pressure centers in the foot, which then provide stimulation to the autonomic and sensory motor nervous systems.

Numerous studies on the therapeutic effects of foot reflexology have and are being done (Kunz, 1999). An American study published in *Obstetrics and Gynecology* demonstrated the effective use of foot reflexology for premenstrual syndrome (Oleson and Flocco, 1993). Nursing studies have been conducted on the effectivity of reflexology for childbirth, urinary retention, neck muscle tension, cystic fibrosis, anxiety levels in the elderly, bowel function, and comforting hospice patients. The Chinese government has published multiple studies on the effective use of reflexology in lowering blood sugar levels in type II diabetics.

Nurses in Switzerland and the United Kingdom are taught foot reflexology as part of their training. "Reflexology is an exciting, absorbing way of introducing new methods of patient care and its use presents many opportunities for nursing research. Because it is so deceptively simple it is important that its potential is not dismissed" (Lockett, 1992, p. 15). Some nurses are already using foot reflexology and receiving insurance reimbursement for it. The January 1995 issue of the New York State Nursing Association Newsletter stated that a clinical nurse oncologist had hospital privileges to treat terminal cancer patients with reflexology (Goldstein, p. 25). She said that she had reduced narcotic interventions for pain control, had documented the effects of reflexology, and that she receives insurance reimbursement for the type of care she provides.

I have integrated reflexology into my nursing practice for fifteen years. Most of my work has not been in the hospital setting although I have had a number of occasions in the hospital setting when I have had patients inadvertently say to me that they wished their "reflexologist was there to help them." One man I took care of, who expressed his wish for his reflexologist, had just had part of a lung removed. He was very uncomfortable with his chest tube. Every time he would move, the chest tube was irritating, even with pain medication. I told him that I was a reflexologist and would give him a gentle foot treatment that might help him to relax. After the footwork, he fell fast asleep for three hours. I have also used reflexology during patients' footbaths, which is a good time to use foot reflexology techniques, especially if the patient is elderly or feels tenderness in the feet. The warm water helps the patient relax and the points being touched on the feet are not as sensitive.

MASSAGE

Massage has been used for centuries throughout the world. There are numerous types of massage: Swedish, osteopathic, neuropathic, shiatsu and Chinese tui na, to name a few. Some of the purposes of massage are organization of the nervous system, deep relaxation, and providing the body the opportunity, through deep relaxation, to reach greater balance and homeostasis between the neuromuscular system and the internal organs. "The sensory information from massage comes through nerve receptors in the skin and muscles (the effect on veins and lymphatic vessels is mechanical). If the massage is perceived as gentle, loving and caring, the limbic system sends this message to the hypothalamus which sets a tone for relaxation and rebalance and healing" (Duggan & Duggan, 1989, p. 30).

The skeletal muscles make up about 40 percent of the human body and therefore their need for oxygen is considerable. When a muscle becomes tense, or contracted, it is no longer able to receive the same amount of blood or oxygen as when it is relaxed. Muscles become inefficient when they are contracted all the time. In the dance world, we call this state of continued inefficient contraction muscular "cement." People who walk around with high levels of continuous stress often exhibit symptoms of muscular cement. It is often difficult for them to lie in a bed and relax because their muscles and nervous systems are in a fixed state of reaction and readiness for activity or stress. Their bodies can become more rigid and less able to take part in nonverbal communication. "It is through the neuromuscular system that we act out our humanity and our individual personalities in the infinite variety of ways of being human . . . it is through our musculoskeletal systems that we act out and communicate our attitudes, fears, hopes, aspirations, beliefs and childhood conditioning" (Duggan & Duggan, 1989, pp. 43–44).

Massage provides care to the musculoskeletal system. It stimulates the flow of blood and lymph fluid. The movement of lymph fluid is dependent upon muscle movement, which is extremely important to the effectiveness of the immune system. Massage is helpful for all excretory functions including lymph drainage. Not so long ago, American physicians used massage in the treatment of illness. It remains a part of medical treatment today in many countries.

The six basic techniques in massage that have been used historically are effleurage, friction, petrissage, tapotement, and vibration. Effleurage, which is defined as gentle strokes used without friction or pressure, is used for relaxation. This is the type of massage stroke taught historically in nursing programs. Friction is a slightly deeper form of massage in which the palms and fingers are used. Petrissage is another name for kneading, as though the muscles were bread dough. The nurse must be trained to pull and knead the tissues without pinching or poking. Tapotement is the same as percussion. I have had babies with chronic lung disease go to sleep during their rhythmic percussion treatment. Tapotement is done with a cupped hand or with the hand used in a chopping fashion. Vibration is used to rapidly shake out a limb or tissue to encourage relaxation.

Relaxation is very difficult for some people. Often people are not aware that they are tensing a muscle when they are not using it. By the nurse touching the tensed area alone, the patient is often able to focus her mind on the body part needing relaxation. Because the mind is usually disconnected from the stress in the body part, asking the patient to "relax" that body part is not helpful. In fact, I make it a point *not* to ask a patient to "relax." The command to "relax" usually causes them to tense more. They say, "What, I'm not relaxed?" I ask them to breathe into the area of the body instead as if able to fill it like a balloon. Or I might ask them to wiggle the area themselves. This facilitates a reconnection of the mind to the tension-filled body part so that the patient can receive the full benefit of massage.

Patients must be involved in the relaxation process. A massage, or any type of touch therapy, is not as effective without the patient's active, and relaxed, participation. "Ideally, the area to be massaged should be unclothed and free of restrictions, while the rest of the body remains draped. Oil or lotion is used to lubricate the skin, allowing the strokes to flow smoothly. The environment should be warm and free of drafts. Distractions should be minimal. Music may be used to lessen distraction and to lull the client into a relaxed state. The working surface should be firm to support the body. Hand hygiene includes short fingernails and smooth cuticles and skin" (White, 1988, p. 66).

INFANT MASSAGE

All of the information provided in the previous section on massage is true for the infant. Babies have a great need for help in neuro-motor organization especially as a result of the stress of the birth process. Babies experience regular periods of stress and need help relaxing, too. I teach parents to massage their babies as a way of developing their ability to communicate with their babies nonverbally.

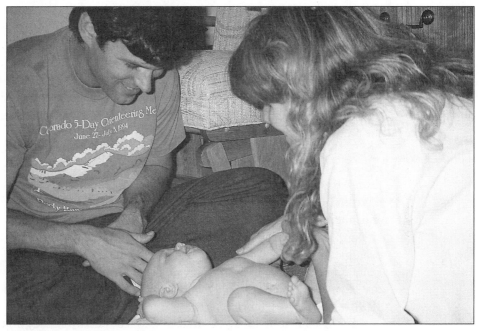

Infant massage

A baby's first communication is touch. They spend nine months in complete contact with the mother's uterus. It is too much to think that babies can give up their touch communication after they are born. The ongoing work of researchers such as Dr. Tiffany Field has shown that premature babies gain weight more steadily when touched (Field & Schanberg, 1986). The brains of babies who are not touched do not develop normally.

Infant massage is healthy touch. Parents who massage their babies teach their children about compassion and love. Nurses must encourage parents to touch their babies and allow them to have skin-to-skin contact with them. There are many parents who have never been the recipients of healthy, intimate, nonsexual touch. Nurses are perfectly positioned to break the cycle of healthy touch deprivation that occurs in some families. Nurses can be teachers of healthy touch.

THERAPEUTIC TOUCH

Therapeutic touch (TT) is a modality developed by Dora Kunz and Delores Krieger. This modality is similar to the laying-on of hands in the sense that the nurse who practices the modality does so to correct and balance disruption in the energy field of the patient. Illness is believed to be the physical manifestation of a disruption in the patient's energy field. The energy field of the body is a scientific concept that will be addressed in greater detail in Chapter 11.

The practice of therapeutic touch has four basic steps: centering, assessment, treatment, and evaluation. The nurse centers herself by sitting in a relaxed position and doing a deep breathing and relaxation exercise that enables her to "experience inner peace and wholeness" (Mackey, 1995, p. 28). The nurse then assesses the patient's energy field with her hands by passing them over the patient's body from head to toe. The nurse then directs energy through her hands, guided by visualization, into the patient's energy field. The intervention is meant to "restore balance to the patient's energy field" (p. 29).

Dr. Janet Quinn, researcher and teacher of therapeutic touch, writes, "Research indicates that TT seems to increase hemoglobin level, induce physiologic relaxation, decrease state anxiety, decrease pain, increase the rate of human wound healing, increase positive affect, including feelings of joy, contentment, vigor, and affection and alter select immunological parameters in both practitioners and recipients" (1992, p. 33). A new study on the use of therapeutic touch for osteoarthritis, for example, found that, ". . . TT decreased arthritis pain, and improved function and general health status in these patients. This improvement was significantly greater than that seen in the placebo group" (Gordon, Merenstein, D'Amico, & Hudgens, 1998, p. 275).

Therapeutic touch is an example of a touch therapy already in use by thousands of nurses. It is a therapy that has helped widen the definition of holistic nursing to include the provision of care that addresses the energetic needs of the patient as well as the bio-psycho-spiritual and social needs.

JIN SHIN JYUTSU

Jin shin is an ancient Japanese hands-on touch modality that also addresses the energy flow of qi (pronounced chee) through the invisible energy channels in the body. Jiro Murai is the Japanese man credited with the discovery of the touch modality jin shin, translated as "the art of the creator through the person of compassion" (Burmeister & Monte, 1997).

This modality is based on the belief that the practitioner, using ancient directions for hand placement, can direct the patient's energy flow through various organs. It is believed that organ "flows" can become disrupted for many reasons including participating in routine, daily activities and that the disruption of energy flows can lead to illness. Jin shin practitioners are taught the redirection and balancing of these organ flows.

Pulse diagnosis, a practice in Eastern medicine, is performed to determine which organ flows are in need of strengthening and balancing. The nurse places her fingertips on the patient's body points as instructed by the manuscript of organ flows originally recorded by Jiro Murai. She keeps her fingertips on the points until the two points, one for each hand, are balanced and in sync. The ability to sense this balancing of pulses is taught by an experienced practitioner. Patients describe the modality as deeply relaxing and refreshing as well as healing. There are different flows for various conditions from fever to heart attack in addition to specific organ flows.

I have used jin shin in practice as a complementary modality for many health care situations. I have used it as an adjunctive therapy with people going through a traumatic procedure, as well as a preventive care modality that people can request as they might request a massage. Anecdotally, many patients having jin shin in addition to biomedical treatments have experienced shorter recovery times. Jin shin, and all the touch therapies, are excellent adjunctive modalities that are noninvasive and complementary to most of the biomedical procedures patients might be engaged in.

Conclusion

Meeting the patient's need for touch is vital to their healing and health care experience. As Montagu says, "The laying on of hands has for centuries been well understood in religious communion. It would be well if it were similarly understood within the healing community. Interestingly enough, the one branch of the healing community, which has recognized the importance of touch, is the nursing profession. Being so much closer to the patient than the doctor, nurses have been in far better position to appreciate the importance of touching in the care of the patient" (1986, p. 282). Nurses must continue to research the therapeutic value of what occurs when they provide the experience of touch to a patient. There is tremendous opportunity to develop and expand the use of touch as a fundamental caring modality in nursing practice. Resources for further learning about touch therapies are provided in Appendix B.

References

Burmeister, A., & Monte, T. (1997). *The touch of healing: Energizing body, mind, and spirit with the art of Jin Shin Jyutsu.* New York: Bantam Books.

Donahue, M. (1996). *Nursing: The finest art* (2nd ed.). St. Louis, MO: Mosby–Yearbook, Inc.

Duggan, J., & Duggan, S. (1989). *Edgar Cayce's massage, hydrotherapy and healing oils.* Virginia Beach, VA: Inner Vision.

Estabrooks, C. (1987). Touch in nursing practice: A historical perspective. *Journal of Nursing History, 2* (2), 33–49.

Field, T. M., & Schanberg, S. M. et al. (1986). Effects of tactile/kinesthetic stimulation on preterm neonates. *Pediatrics, 77* (5), 654–658.

Fitzgerald, W. H., & Bowers, E. F. (1917). *Zone therapy.* Columbus, OH: I.W. Long.

Goldstein, F. (1995). Mind-body spirit: Are all three needed in the healing process? *New York State Nursing Association Newsletter,* Jan./Feb., 25.

Gordon, A., Merenstein, J., D'Amico, F., & Hudgens, D. (1998). The effects of therapeutic touch on patients with osteoarthritis of the knee. *The Journal of Family Practice, 47* (4), 271–277.

Kunz, B., &. Kunz, K. (1999). *Medical applications of reflexology: Findings in research about safety, efficacy, mechanism of action and cost-effectiveness of reflexology.* Albuquerque, NM: Reflexology Research.

Lawless, J. (1998). *Aromatherapy and the mind.* London: Thorsons.

Lockett, J. (1992). Reflexology—Nursing tool? *Australian Nurses Journal, 22* (1), 14–15.

Mackey, R. (1995). Discover the healing power of therapeutic touch. *American Journal of Nursing,* 27–32.

McClelland, D., & Kirshnit, C. (1988). The effect of motivational arousal through films on salivary immunoglobulin. *Psychology and Health, 2,* 31–52.

Montagu, A. (1986). *Touching: The human significance of the skin* (3rd ed.). New York: Harper & Row.

Mower, M. (1997). Massage returns to nursing. *Massage Magazine,* Sept./Oct. (69), 47–54.

Mulaik, J., Megenity, J., Cannon, R., Chance, K., Cannella, K., Garland, L., & Gilead, M. (1991). Patients' perceptions of nurses' use of touch. *Western Journal of Nursing Research, 13* (3), 306–323.

Oleson, T., & Flocco, W. (1993). Randomized controlled study of premenstrual symptoms treated with ear, hand and foot reflexology. *Obstetrics and Gynecology, 82* (6), 906–911.

Quinn, J. (1992). The senior's therapeutic touch education program. *Holistic Nursing Practice, 7* (1), 32–37.

Routasalo, P., & Lauri, S. (1996). Developing an instrument for the observation of touching. *Clinical Nurse Specialist, 10* (6), 293–299.

Weinrich, S., & Weinrich, M. (1990). The effect of massage on pain in cancer patients. *Applied Nursing Research, 3* (4), 140–145.

White, J. (1988). Touching with intent: Therapeutic massage. *Holistic Nursing Practice, 2* (3), 63–67.

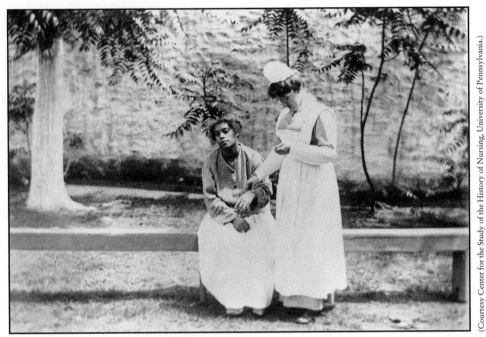

The healing force of nature

Never go to a doctor whose office plants have died.

—ERMA BOMBECK

CHAPTER 8

Creating a Healing Environment Within and Without

The History of Nursing and the Healing Environment

Nightingale's statement about "putting the patient in the best condition possible for nature to work upon him" implies that the patient and "nature" have a relationship. It also implies that nature has the ability to heal. Nightingale knew that humans have the ability to heal from within and without. People have within them what she called a "vital power" that sustains them. This vital power of nature, and in nature, is the energy of healing that nurses witness in their intimate daily work with patients.

This vital power is present and at work in the inner "environment" of the patient. It is present in the outer environment surrounding and influencing the patient. Florence Nightingale based her nursing practice upon a belief and knowledge in the vital power within the patient and environment. "It [nursing practice] ought to signify the proper use of fresh air, light, warmth, cleanliness, quiet and the proper selection and administration of diet—all at the least expense of vital power to the patient" (Nightingale, 1957, p. 6). Nightingale's book, *Notes on Nursing,* covers each of these environmental topics in detail.

Although very little has been written on the importance of environment to nursing practice since the time of Nightingale, common sense tells us that the effect of the patient's environment, both internal and external, is of vital importance to health. This chapter discusses the second category of caring modalities used throughout history as a way nurses demonstrate caring—creating a healing environment.

EXTERNAL ENVIRONMENT

The nurse ensures a healthy external environment for patients. "The nurse must see that his [the patient's] physical environment is conducive to recovery. The room should be simply and attractively furnished with appointments which enable the attending physician and nurse to give the necessary care to the patient with the minimum of demands upon his strength. . . . Temperature, humidity and ventilation are important factors to be considered. . . . A room which is quiet and has a pleasant outlook contributes to the mental comfort of the patient" (Tracy, 1938, p. 31). The nurse must be aware of the importance of the patient's environment because of its impact on the health of a patient. "We take our everyday physical milieu for granted most of the time; nevertheless, we cherish its familiarity. The effect of physical space can be seen in everyday situations" (Cumming & Cumming, 1962, p. 89).

Nurses must be aware of the patient's need for environmental familiarity, their own need for familiarity, and how these two needs interact. For example, nurses are often asked to "float" to another department to care for patients. The nurse can easily become stressed because she is not in her usual environment. This may affect her ability to provide the best care to the patient.

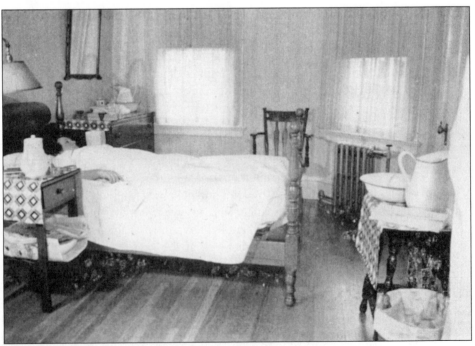

The healing home environment, 1938 *(From Margaret Tracy,* Nursing: An Art and a Science. *St. Louis, MO: The C.V. Mosby Company, 1938. Used with permission.)*

Patients experience the same kind of stress in the unfamiliar surroundings of a hospital. They are out of their element and often talk about going home to "their own bed" and how good that will feel. I have often heard patients say that they "go to hospitals and doctors' offices for treatment but they go home to heal." As both Nightingale and Tracy point out so clearly, the nurse's job is to create an environment that does not tax the strength or vital power the patient needs for healing. It is a challenge for nurses to be creative and find ways to overcome the obvious obstacles to the patient's healing such as being in an unfamiliar environment.

Today, many nurses participate in creating a healing environment to meet patient and staff needs. One example of an organization that focuses on the environmental experience of the patient is a health care organization called Planetree. Planetree was founded in 1978 by Angelica Thierot with the purpose of creating health facilities that "empower patients emphasizing patient involvement, patient education, and provide a healing, home-like atmosphere" (Moore & Komras, 1993, pp. 3–4).

As we begin the new millennium, the need for nurses to focus on the importance of a healing environment becomes imperative. Environmental stressors upon patients and the staff caring for them are great. As technology continues to advance, and high-tech environments become more prominent in health care, the need for nurses to assist patients in creating a balanced environment that addresses the needs of the body, mind, and spirit is important. Nurses can be taught how to do this. "The nursing arts laboratory of the 21st century may engage students in the examination of color, architecture, and other features of the aesthetic environment that may influence the quality of client interactions" (Smith, 1994, p. 7).

The nurse and his behaviors are also part of the patient's "environment." The nurse is not just existing *in* the patient's environment; he can also *be* a healing environment for the patient. Dr. Janet Quinn writes, "If I *am* the healing environment for this client, how can I *be* a more healing environment? How can I become a safe space, a sacred healing vessel for this client in this moment? How can I use my consciousness, my being, my voice, my touch, my face, for healing?" (Quinn, 1992, p. 27). Historical nursing texts project a vision of the nurse creating and being in the healing environment. Writers such as Nightingale, Henderson, and Tracy all discuss in detail the way to enter a patient's room and how to *be* with patients. For example, Nightingale writes, "Apprehension, uncertainty, waiting, expectation, fear of surprise do a patient more harm than any exertion. . . . Always tell a patient and tell him beforehand when you are going out and when you will be back, whether it is a day, an hour or ten minutes" (Nightingale, 1957, p. 22). This is just one example of the importance of the nurse as being both a part of the patient's environment and being in the patient's environment. The nurse enhances the healing relationship with the patient by understanding his needs for the familiarity and security of his environment.

As we look to the future of the healing environment, we can see that places such as Planetree hospitals that provide homelike environments may be better able to address patients' environmental needs, including sensory experiences, security, and familiarity to help them feel comforted and cared for. Hospitals just might "become temples of healing, where form follows function and the sacred art of healing joins with the modern miracle of medical technology" (Moore & Komras, 1993, p. 179).

INTERIOR ENVIRONMENT

Throughout most of recent history, medicine's view of disease has been that it is caused by an external "intruder," such as bacteria or a virus. Florence Nightingale did not agree. She believed that diseases were conditions that the nurse and patient had control over. Nightingale said, "Is it not living in a continual mistake to look upon diseases, as we do now, as separate entities, which must exist, like cats and dogs? Instead of looking upon them as conditions, like a dirty and clean condition, and just as much under our own control; or rather as the reactions of kindly nature, against the conditions in which we have placed ourselves. For disease, as all experience shows, are adjectives, not noun substantives" (Nightingale, 1957, p. 19). Nursing care clearly affects the outcome of disease. A nurse's keen attention to the environment and lifestyle of a patient often reveal the contributors to the patient's diseased state. Nightingale showed nurses what this was all about when she appeared at the side of the soldiers at the Crimea. She observed her patients and found ways to improve their care by creating a healthy environment.

Research of scientists such as German bacteriologist Dr. Guenther Enderlein have shed more light on Nightingale's statement that diseases are conditions. Enderlein used dark field microscopy in which a specimen is illuminated against a dark background by a special condenser that provides light at a 45 degree angle. With the aid of the superior images from the microscope, he found that microorganisms live in a symbiotic relationship in the body in a nonharmful form he called the protit phase. They inhabit the blood, body fluids, and different cell tissues. He found that, "Under certain conditions, the microorganisms can lose their symbiotic qualities and evolve through different stages into other forms and sizes, literally growing hostile and able to destroy surrounding tissue cells. This primarily takes place when the body suffers a significant change in milieu, becoming more alkaline or acidic" (Enby, 1990, p. 25). Although Enderlein agreed that commonly held scientific beliefs founded upon the research of Pasteur were "partially" true of specific infectious diseases caused by certain bacteria and virus, they were not sufficient to explain noncontagious diseases such as chronic illness.

I worked with a physician who showed me the protits Enderlein spoke about. We used a microscope attached to a large viewing screen to examine blood samples from patients. The physician monitored changes in the "inner environment" of the patient after prescribing diet changes, medications or supplements, and other health treatments to bring about greater balance. We were able to watch the changes occurring in the patients' inner environments following treatment.

Nurses recognize the need of the patient for greater balance, homeostasis, and adaptation and, therefore, are involved in assisting patients to make changes in their interior "environment," exterior "environment," or both. Nurses do this by facilitating lifestyle changes. In working with patients I first explain the importance of a balanced lifestyle. I suggest to the patient the image of a scale, the old kind with two shallow dishes hanging from the ends of a pole. I explain that when all aspects of their life, food choices, relationships, spiritual connection, activity, rest, housing, and work, are in balance, relative to their personal needs, the "scales" are balanced. When some change occurs in any of these life areas, the scales are tipped, and the health of the patient depends on their ability to adapt, or rebalance the scales.

Life is in a constant state of movement and balance between excesses and deficiencies of all kinds. Many people are aware of the old adage, "everything in moderation." This is a statement about balance. Nurses often enter healing relationships with patients whose scales are tipped, either due to excesses or deficiencies of some kind or another. For example, I have often worked with depressed patients who are *deficient* in sleep. Sometimes an antidepressant medication or counseling is the best remedy for their suffering. But sometimes helping the patient explore ways to improve sleep reveals simple health solutions that can make a tremendous difference. I once found that a patient only needed to develop a bedtime ritual of self-care that included a hot bath and a warm beverage. His ability to sleep improved and the depression improved as well.

Another example of the patient needing help with balancing lifestyle is the patient addicted to alcohol. This patient takes in *too much* of a substance that in smaller quantities can be medicinal. The alcoholic is out of balance due to *excess* alcohol and his *choice* to drink the alcohol in excess. The patient has a problem of "excess" both physically and mentally.

The goal in both cases of deficiency and excess is to assist the patient in learning ways to maintain balance as life changes occur. Helping patients work with the concept of balance in lifestyle and health is an ongoing process. It is a process that challenges all the patient's internal and external means of adaptation. Much of what integrative nurses do in putting the patient in the best condition possible for nature to work upon them is to creatively support the adaptation process.

The concept of adaptation is not new to nursing. Nurse theorist Sister Callista Roy wrote a nursing practice model called "The Adaptation Model." One of the major concepts of the nursing model is that the environment, which is "the world within and around the person," stimulates the patient's ability to make an "adaptive response." "As the environment changes, the person has the opportunity to continue to grow and develop and to enhance the meaning of life for self and others. The environment includes all conditions, circumstances, and influences surrounding and affecting the development and behavior of the person" (Roy & Andrews, 1986, pp. 7–8).

The environment, both within and without, has a profound effect upon the health of patients and their ability to cope with and adapt to new situations. The nurse's role in the health care environment is to creatively and scientifically explore the many ways changes in that environment can demonstrate caring to patients. The nurse-artist's palette is full to overflowing with opportunities to regulate environmental changes, by increasing or decreasing warmth, coolness, air, sound, smells, water, plants, animals, people, energy, and light. Nurses need to just pick up the "paintbrush" and continue exploring the many ways subtle changes in the environment within and without can promote healing and health.

The Art and Science of Demonstrating Care by Creating a Healing Environment

Creating a healing environment takes scientific as well as aesthetic skill. Historically, the concept of creating a healing environment has been prominent in the nursing care provided in inpatient psychiatric facilities. Milieu therapy, creating a therapeutic environment for patients, has been a recognized form of therapy for decades. The literature on milieu therapy reveals some of the importance of environment to the health and well-being of patients.

The main purpose of the physical milieu is to "provide a setting in which the patient is supported by a feeling of familiarity and continuity" (Cumming & Cumming, 1962, pp. 102–103). In addition, the patient is oriented to space and time by the physical cues provided in the environment. These cues must be as specific to the patient's cultural identity as possible. "When physical cues are present, but ambiguous, they lead to disrupted ego feeling, disorientation, and anxiety. . . . There is evidence that any change requiring ego reorganization will bring about some set dedifferentiation and diffusion feeling, resulting in a change in self concept or orientation to self. It is a common phenomenon, for example, to hear people express new ideas about themselves after their first serious illness in adult life" (p. 93).

Patients need to look at themselves in the mirror, and not just to see how they look to others. They need to see their own face to help them orient to person. A person's own face is most familiar to them. It is compassionate care that nurses provide when they encourage a patient to look at himself in the mirror, or encourage family members to bring in familiar objects from home for the hospitalized patient. Patients who have familiar objects around them, especially when they are given medications (such as narcotics) that can alter their perceptions, are less likely to spend their vital power on orienting themselves to their surroundings and decreasing the anxiety they feel in an unfamiliar space. They can use their vital power for healing.

Patients need to be oriented to self, place, and time. Many things can happen to people who are ill that pose a challenge to their ability to maintain a sense of who and where they are. Patients need to know the time and date. Part of having a strong sense of self is being able to anticipate the future. Patients who do not know what time it is often experience anxiety or discomfort. I have taken care of women who have had to be hospitalized for weeks with bedrest orders to protect the babies growing inside them. These mothers often meticulously keep calendars and schedules so that they can maintain some sense of order and orientation about their days in the hospital.

Maintaining order in an environment is important to the care of patients. Order means familiarity. Think of the blind patient who is completely independent in an environment they have organized and memorized. If furniture is moved, the blind patient begins to bump into things and feels anxious about his ability to care for himself. It is no different for the person who is not blind.

The human brain is "wired" to identify the familiar and the unfamiliar. The fight or flight response can be activated by the unfamiliar environment. "Proshansky, Ittleson and Rivlin (1976) observed that individuals attempt to organize their physical environment so that their freedom of choice is maximized. When people feel unable to control their situation, they may feel angry with themselves and the 'system,' feel humiliated and degraded, and express low self-worth and self-esteem. When people cannot choose and are bothered by their environment, the consequences may be negative for their health. Brown (1987) found empowering environments were more pleasant, made the actors feel good about themselves and others, and were related to manifestations of greater human well-being and productivity" (Davidson, 1988, pp. 36–37).

Most people take their environments for granted and are oblivious to them. It is when something changes that they sense and experience their environment with full conscious awareness. Nurses can use temperature, sound, light, color, and physical aspects of the patient's environment to provide familiarity, continuity, order, and peace to patients.

The Environment and Integrative Nursing

Many of the concepts of environmental intervention written about by Florence Nightingale are still appropriate for today's nurse. Nurses deal with many of the same issues of noise, temperature, order, and cleanliness in the environment that were encountered by the nurses of the 1800s. This section discusses some of the creative ways nurses deal with meeting the sensory needs of patients through environmental change. This section also includes the historical and conventional ways of using environmental substances such as water and plants to address patient needs for comfort and care. Although they are indeed part of the creation of a healing environment, the therapeutic use of light and energy will be dealt with separately in Chapter 11.

SOUND AND SLEEP

Sound is a common occurrence in any environment. Sound can be pleasant or disturbing to patients especially as they convalesce. Noise is defined as disturbing sound that is "unnecessary and creates an expectation in the mind of the patient" (Nightingale, 1957, p. 25). A nurse often becomes the advocate for control of noise in the environment because of her knowledge of the importance of a patient's ability to rest and sleep.

Many patients find the ability to rest and sleep troublesome during illness. They often suffer from pain or mental distress that keeps them from experiencing a rest that leaves them feeling refreshed and strengthened. This phenomenon is complicated by the activities going on in their environment especially when they are hospitalized. Patients are disturbed by lights being turned on and off, nurses taking vital signs and doing procedures, and unfamiliar noise in the hallways and in their rooms. One study by Woods in 1972 documented fifty-six interruptions of sleep on the first postoperative night for cardiac patients (Southwell & Wistow, 1995, p. 1102).

Sleep is considered by many nurses to be the most important factor in the body's ability to restore itself. Yet many patients suffer from sleep deprivation while in the care of nurses. Rest and sleep are both critical to the patient's ability to heal. Research shows that there is an increased need for sleep during stress and illness (Southwell & Wistow, 1995, p. 1102).

The study, by Southwell and Wistow, showed that patients and nurses had different opinions as to what noises caused patients to get less sleep. Nurses "reported less frequently than patients on the noises from their own behavior, in particular the noises arising from talking to each other and from their shoes . . . nurses perceived some activities associated with their work to be more disruptive than was reported by patients, for example fetching commodes or bedpans, giving treatments and talking to patients" (1995, p. 1107). It is interesting to note that patients did not perceive nurses' *caring* behaviors to be disruptive to sleep.

Nowadays, physicians routinely place standing orders for sleeping pills for their patients in the hope of ensuring a good sleep; the pills do not always work. Hypnotics were used in the early part of the century, as well, but only after "all preparations for sleep were completed. . . . Doctors will quickly come to recognize the nurses who have used their skill in nursing care before requesting such orders" for sleeping pills (Tracy, 1938, p. 112). Historically some of the interventions used by nurses to help a patient sleep were hot milk or broth, back rubs, talking about the patient's worries, and positioning. It was thought that raising the head of the bed would decrease circulation to the head and the patient would be less apt to have recurrent thoughts to keep him awake. Tracy also writes that, "If a sick patient has complete confidence in his nurse, he will be more apt to drop off to sleep, because he feels assured that he will be well cared for as he sleeps" (p. 112).

The more care is demonstrated by nurses during a patient's waking hours, the more confident the patient will feel when he sleeps that the nurse will be there if needed. I have seen this to be especially true with young children in the hospital. They sleep much more soundly if their parent is at the bedside and they have gotten to know the nurse who cares for them. Nurses must continue to evaluate whether the benefits of the caring interventions they perform on behalf of the patient, and which sometimes waken the patient, outweigh those of undisturbed sleep.

Just as sleep is a change in the body's energy flow or rhythm, so is sound or noise in the environment a change in rhythm. "Smith (1986) studied rest as 'the person's experience of easing with the flow of rhythmic change in the environment.' Her findings suggested that random, unstructured noise in a supposedly quiet environment promoted tension and irritability. A patterned auditory input of sound contributed to easing with the flow of the environment" (Davidson, 1988, p. 36). One form of patterned sound is music.

Music has proved to be helpful in creating a healing environment for some patients. Throughout history, rhythm and music have been used to enhance the healing process. The Greek philosopher Pythagoras often *prescribed* music to help "maintain harmony of the body and soul" (Olson, 1998, p. 569). "Since rhythm does have such a definite effect upon the body, the ancient Indians, Greeks and Egyptians and American Indians, we know, were very careful as to the use and kind of rhythmic music taught to children. They all realized that the irritation caused by discordant rhythms in the delicate constitution of a child would cause bursts of temper and serious ills of both body and mind" (Retallack, 1973, pp. 62–63).

Studies have shown that music has tremendous influence on many disease states such as anxiety, pain, nausea due to chemotherapy, and memory loss, to name a few. Music has been helpful in elder care as well. Joan, in her narrative in Chapter 4, discussed how she used music in the care of an elderly German woman at a nursing home. The woman spoke no English and rarely interacted with anyone. Joan made a tape of German folksongs and brought it to the home one day to play it for the woman. The woman cried and sang and was happier than she had been in months. Music can be integrated into the plan of care for all patients, from neonates to seniors.

VENTILATION, BREATHING, AND TEMPERATURE

Florence Nightingale taught the importance of fresh air. She said to "keep the air as pure as possible without chilling the patient" (Nightingale, 1957, p. 8). In Chinese and Ayurvedic (Indian) medicine, it is believed that fresh air contains vital energy that stimulates the body's own vital power. In China the vital energy is called qi (pronounced chee) and in India it is called prana. In most hospitals in the United States, windows do not open. All air goes through an internal ventilation system. I have often wondered if Nightingale was so vehement about opening the windows and fresh air because she had knowledge of this vital force in the air. It has been believed for centuries that the humidity, temperature, and movement of the air all affect the health of

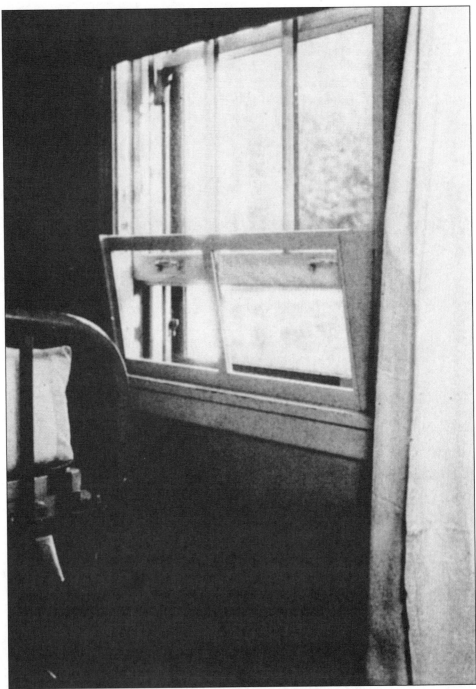

Window ventilator, 1938 (*From Margaret Tracy,* Nursing: An Art and a Science. *St. Louis, MO: The C.V. Mosby Company, 1938. Used with permission.*)

the patient. It is the job of the nurse to find the temperature of a room and air quality that does not significantly tax the patient's energy, which he needs for healing. A patient who is cold or having difficulty breathing in a stuffy room spends much energy trying to breathe and keep warm and spends less energy on healing. "Sanitarians have come to regard an abundant supply of pure fresh air, well conditioned, as one of the real essentials for health and maximum efficiency. Circulating air of proper temperature and moisture carries off body heat and contributes to comfort" (Tracy, 1938, p. 33). Hence the importance of having healing facilities that allow the regulation of fresh air and temperature to the individual needs of patients.

Patients experience air and temperature changes through breathing as well as through the skin. Breathing is vital to life. Breathing can enhance the adaption to one's environment. Instructing patients to perform consciously controlled breathing has been used as a caring modality of obstetrical nursing for decades. Nurses know that women who use breathing techniques during labor have less pain and anxiety and are better able to focus on their bodies during the birth process. Conscious breathing is also part of meditation and yoga practices used in stress reduction and lifestyle change programs such as Dr. Jon Kabat-Zinn's program, Stress Reduction and Relaxation, at the University of Massachusetts Medical Center.

Breath is the physical reminder of the vital power. Breathing occurs whether we think of it or not. When we actively and consciously focus on breathing we enter the realm of the vital power. Breath is life. Candice Pert writes that, "There is a wealth of data showing that changes in the rate and depth of breathing produce changes in the quality and kind of peptides that are released from the brainstem. The peptide-respiratory link is well documented: Virtually any peptide found anywhere else can be found in the respiratory center. This peptide substrate may provide the scientific rationale for the powerful healing effects of consciously controlled breathing patterns" (Pert, 1997, pp. 186–187). Perhaps scientific discovery is finally catching up to what Nightingale knew and practiced all along.

PLANT USE IN NURSING

Throughout the history of nursing, in fact until only about fifty years ago, plant medicines were routinely used and administered by nurses. Before the significant growth of the pharmaceutical industry after World War II, most medications used in healing practices were derived from plants. Most medications, except for narcotics, were sold over the counter and many households practiced "domestic medical practice," or self-medication and treatment, which included the use of plants for healing. I received a book from a retired American nurse called, *Domestic Medical Practice: A Household Advisor in the Treatment of Diseases Arranged for Family Use,* an eight-inch-thick tome filled with the medical knowledge of the early 1900s, which was used by the nurse's family for decades. The chapter on nursing care discusses plant medicines and their internal and external use.

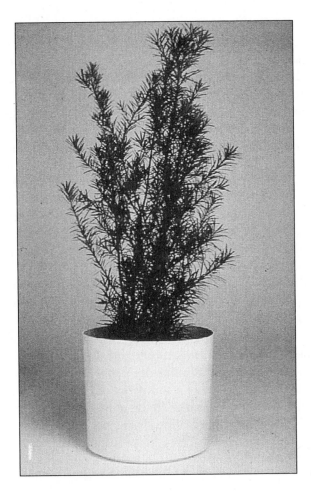

Courtesy H. Edward Reiley.

Twenty-five percent of the prescriptions written in the United States from 1959 to 1980 contained plant extracts or an active principle prepared from a plant (Farnsworth, Akerele, Bingel, Soejarto, & Guo, 1985, p. 966). The World Health Organization has estimated that 80 percent of the world's population continues to rely upon traditional medicines such as plant-derived medicines for their health care needs. Plant or herbal medicine is not new to communities who practice self-care nor is it new to nursing practice. It is only since biomedical science began to focus on the development of pharmaceutical drugs and the germ theory that plant medicines fell out of use among physicians and nurses as well. Just because physicians in the West no longer prescribe plant medicines and topical applications does not mean that the public has forgotten or stopped using these time-honored remedies and comfort measures.

An American nursing study on the self-care practices of patients using botanical remedies showed that "most respondents judged their home remedies to be helpful"

(Brown & Marcy, 1991, p. 348). They write that, "The figures on use of botanicals obtained in this study are doubtless inexact. Still they illustrate how firmly entrenched self-care is in American culture and how persistently unorthodox therapies survive, even among Americans with access to conventional healthcare. . . . Knowledge of this lay perspective and self care activities should aid diagnosis of the individual patient's needs and resources before initiating an intervention" (p. 348).

Although I agree with the investigators that it is imperative that nurses understand people's health care and self-care practices, I do not agree that the use of plant medicines is unorthodox in the least. It is in fact a vital part of vernacular, or common everyday, healing practices. Herbs such as coffee and various teas are used every day in many households. Plant use in Western cultural practice and tradition lives on despite the boom in pharmaceutical science and products.

One nurse educator writes about her encouragement of students exploring the self-care practices of their own culture as well as that of their patients. "The most popular topic students chose reflect uses of special foods, herbs, teas and other substance ingested in the belief that they are healthful" (Dehn, 1990, p. 13). One example of common plant medicine practice the students found was the use of topical applications of plant medicines.

The use of aloe vera was a common finding. Aloe has been used medicinally at least since Biblical times. Aloe, along with many other herbs and healing plants and trees, is mentioned in the Bible. It has been used topically for burns and more recently has been integrated into the practice of burn centers. One study from the University of Chicago Burn Center found aloe vera to be "therapeutically beneficial in a burn wound" (Robson, Heggers, & Hagstrom, 1982, p. 162). They found aloe vera to have an anesthetic, broad-spectrum antimicrobial effect, and an antithromboxane effect. They also found that aloe vera is rich in fatty acids, which they hypothesized supply the nutrients necessary for maturation of healthy tissue.

Aloe vera is only one of the many plant substances used historically as topical remedies. Onions, garlic, flaxseed, linseed, bran, mustard, and hops were applied as packs, poultices, plasters, ointments, liniments, therapeutic baths, or oils. The poultice was one of the most common tratments until the time of Pasteur and Lister and was used for ailments such as pleuritis, pneumonia, bronchitis, enteritis, hepatitis, and peritonitis. Cold poultices were used for ulcers, gangrene, and after amputations (Haller, 1985).

Nurses were well versed in the therapeutic actions of plants. As the retired nurses stated in their narratives in Chapter 4, they had to know the category of action for each plant medicine so that they would understand the therapy. They learned which plant medicines had astringent, tonic, stimulant, sedative, antispasmodic, alterative, emetic, cathartic, laxative, diuretic, purgative, expectorant, inhalation, emmenagogue, and counter-irritant action. It is no different from today's nursing student learning pharmaceutical classifications of drugs such as beta-blockers, anticholinergics, or antipsychotics.

Plants such as mustard and capsicum (hot pepper) were well known for their counter-irritant action. Parker writes, "Counterirritants are therapeutic agents applied to the skin for the purpose of relieving some deep-seated affection. Counter-irritation relieves the affection of the organ over which it is applied by reflex nerve relation between the skin and the organ, and by producing a change in the blood supply of the organ" (1921, p. 264). Capsaicin, the active principle in capsicum, is being sold today in an over-the-counter ointment for arthritis and other pain relief. There are numerous clinical trials that have demonstrated the effectiveness of topical capsaicin for relief of joint pain (Deal et al., 1991; McCarthy & McCarty, 1992; Capsaicin Study Group, 1991). How many nurses learn to recommend capsicum cream for pain relief?

Clay poultices were used frequently by nurses to retain heat and decrease swelling of patients' sore joints. The clay was said to abstract or draw out fluid from the tissues. To receive a clay poultice or bath today a patient must go to a spa such as those in the mountains of Colorado or New Mexico.

The internal use of plant medicines has grown significantly in the past few years in many Western countries. The increasing consumption of herbal teas and supplements by the American public is of continual concern to regulating bodies such as the Food and Drug Administration (FDA). Questions regarding the safety of these plant medicines for self-care are valid. Yet the number of overdose and toxicity cases reported to poison control centers is minimal. Plant medicines continue to be relatively "safe" for intermittent use. My continued concern is that most plant medicines are taken in pill or capsule form rather than decocted, or steeped as tea, or taken in liquid extraction form. The public has been taught that pills are good medicine. In the case of pharmaceutical drugs, maybe. But this is not necessarily so in the case of plant medicines. Not all plant medicines are meant to be eaten.

SAFETY.   Safety in plant medicine use begins with the recognition of the plant. When I studied Chinese herbal medicine, I was tested on recognition of over two hundred plants in their natural and dried state. The plant medicine practitioner strives to properly identify, and even grow, the plants used in practice. Often, patients have no idea of the origin of the plant medicine they are taking, what it tastes like, or how it affects the body.

Historically, people had more knowledge of plant remedies, as well as a wisdom about plant use, that was passed down from generation to generation, frequently through the women of the family. This is no longer the dominant way people learn about plant medicines in the West. As a result, many consumers are conflicted about the use of plant medicines. They want to learn about the benefits of plant medicines because they know that pharmaceutical drugs often have side effects and do not provide relief in all situations. Many people are aware of the problems biomedical practitioners face regarding the numerous drug-drug and drug-food interactions. In April 1998, *Lancet* reported that dose-dependent adverse drug reactions were the fourth leading cause of death in the United States (Bonn, 1998).

Patients often believe that plant medicine is safer to use because it is in a more natural state. They may also believe that because their grandmother took a particular plant medicine it is safe for them. In moderate amounts, this may be true. But, our grandmothers were not taking the amount of pharmaceutical drugs that the elderly of today are taking, and the physical environment and our bodies have changed very much as society has become more "advanced." Just as patients react differently to drugs, they also react differently to plant medicines, even those plants that are from very pure sources.

In explaining safety of plant medicines to patients, I often use the analogy of the apple. I show them an apple and a spoonful of crystallized fructose that looks like sugar. I tell them I understand that they believe that it is safer for them to eat the apple (the plant medicine) than one of the active ingredients in the apple, the fructose (the pharmaceutical drug). Then I remind them that some plant medicines can cause harm to certain people. For instance, some people have allergic reactions to apples. I recommend that if a patient is planning to use the plant medicine for treating a chronic condition (i.e., use the medicine for more than thirty days), they acquire the help of a medical herbalist.

EDUCATION. Nurses can help patients use plant medicines safely by becoming more educated themselves in the science and art of medicinal plant use and by providing referral sources to patients. A guideline for referral to a medical herbalist is available to assist nurses in the referral process (Libster, 1999). One nursing organization that is experienced in the use of specific plant medicines, both for internal and external use, is the Anthroposophical Nursing Society. They routinely provide continuing education to nurses about the use of plants in health care. Anthroposophical nurses use plants topically when providing comfort and healing to patients. Some clinics in Switzerland and England practice the anthroposophical theories of health care. The nurses in these clinics provide patients with treatments such as lemon compresses and chamomile inhalations.

PLANTS IN THE ENVIRONMENT. Plants, in addition to being taken internally, are used for healing in other ways. Many hospitals have built solariums where patients can go to be among the life-giving energy of plants. Duncan Grosart, a horticulturist, describes the ability of plants to make even a hospital environment relaxing and harmonious (1995). In the United States there are graduate programs offered in horticultural therapy, the use of plants as a therapeutic intervention in mental illness. As a clinical herbalist, I have encouraged my clients to grow or pick their remedy directly. As the patient cares for the plant and harvests from it, the patient gets to know the qualities of the plant. The plant's qualities are its "personality." As a person gets to know the plant and its personality, a healing relationship develops with the plant from which they can gain an understanding of the plant's use in their healing process. Just as we "train" our bodies to "ask" for a medication for a particular discomfort by offering the drug, we can "train" our bodies to ask for plant medicines that have helped us in the past. For example, we can sip on feverfew tea or take Tylenol for a headache, whichever our body "asks" for. Nurses are encountering more and more people who have gotten to know the benefits of herbs for certain conditions and who are then able to ask for plant medicines in the same way they might ask for a drug.

Plants also have the ability to cleanse and freshen the environment. Plants have been studied for their ability to remove toxic waste and heavy metals from soil and water, a process called *phytoremediation* (Negri & Hinchman, 1996). Many plants have strong antibacterial, antiviral, and antifungal properties and have the ability to disinfect our environment and minimize the microbial bombardment our patients are exposed to, especially in hospitals. There are many researchers in the United States, Europe, and Asia who are currently studying the health effects of aromatherapy in the creation of a more healthy environment in hospitals.

AROMATHERAPY.   Aromatherapy is the science of using naturally occurring, highly concentrated plant substances, known as essential oils, in the stimulation of the senses to promote healing of body, mind, and spirit. The antimicrobial effects of essential oils, used in the perfume industry, are well known. "It is said that Bucklersbury, England, was spared from plague because it was the center of the lavender trade, and even today the French city of Grasse, where so much perfume is produced, is known for having very low rates of respiratory illness" (Green & Keville, 1995, p. 10). Besides the effects of essential oils on the immune system, essential oils directly affect the central nervous system. "For example, 'euphoric' odors such as clary sage and grapefruit stimulate the thalamus to secrete neurochemicals called enkephalins, natural pain killers that also produce a general feeling of well-being" (p. 9). I have often wondered what it would be like to practice nursing in a health facility where patient's pain was controlled by changes in their environment such as the subtle introduction of grapefruit odor into a patient's room. Fragrances associated with essential oils have been used for the healing of the mind and emotions as well. "Some remedies are effective in the form of an incense, fumigant or inhalant, especially for the treatment of psychological disorders" (Lawless, 1998, p. 19).

As in perfumery, "more" is not better in aromatherapy. There is an art as well as a science to the use of scent and essential oils in healing that must be learned. My first teacher in the use of essential oils for healing was my foot reflexology mentor. We added small amounts of essential oils to a sweet almond oil, the "carrier oil," to make our own massage oils that we then used on the feet of our patients. We used pure essential oil of rose, lavender, eucalyptus, rosemary, melissa, ylang, dill, and peppermint, to name a few. I learned how to formulate my own massage oil blends and how to use the scented oil with massage to enable the patient to experience greater comfort and balance.

Balance is the goal in the use of essential oils. The oils can be energizing, sedating, or somewhere in between when used for patient care. Improper use of an essential oil, such as applying too much on the skin, can be harmful for a particular patient. Aromatherapy is an ancient art and science for which there are many studies that have proved what ancient Egyptians, Greeks, and Romans knew (American Association of Naturopathic Physicians, 1997, pp. 178–181). Aromatherapy can reduce stress, anxiety, pain, and infection as well as enhance mood.

THE THERAPEUTIC USE OF WATER IN NURSING PRACTICE

Hydrotherapy, or the therapeutic use of water, is one of the oldest caring modalities known to man. "As water is the most prevalent substance on earth, it is no surprise that humans have long used water therapeutically. The oldest records describing hydrotherapy methods can be found in 6,000 year-old Sanskrit writings" (American Association of Naturopathic Physicians, 1997, p. 265). Historical textbooks on nursing practice detail the numerous hydrotherapy applications used by nurses for centuries. Nurses were educated in the art and science of water applications for healing disease as well as for providing comfort.

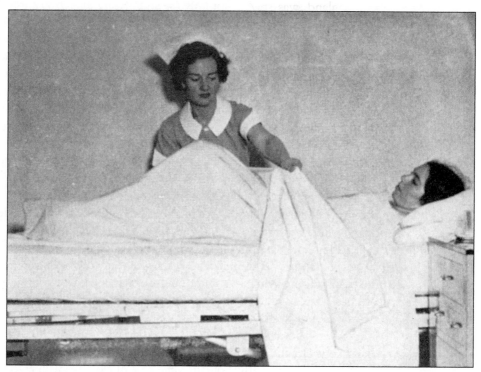

Footbath in bed, 1938 *(From Margaret Tracy,* Nursing: An Art and a Science. *St. Louis, MO: The C.V. Mosby Company, 1938. Used with permission.)*

Water, fresh or salt, hot or cold, played a major role in the care of patients with infectious disease, skin illness, kidney disease, nervous conditions, and almost any malady. Hydrotherapy was a major component of the hands-on work of nurses. Bertha Harmer and Virginia Henderson wrote a textbook outlining the use of baths and packs in hydrotherapy practice. Nurses learned the different uses for full baths, half baths, hot baths, sedative baths, cold baths, continuous baths, saline baths, alcohol baths, alkaline baths, sulfur baths, mustard baths, hot packs, cold packs, sedative packs, and full body sheet packs. Nurses were trained in the proper use of water temperature for affecting certain conditions. They also learned about adding certain substances such as sea salt to the bath to affect body and bath temperature. Baths at body temperature and cold packs were used as sedatives and hot baths and packs were used to increase circulation and to relieve inflammation and congestion of internal organs. "A hot bath that increases perspiration and the elimination of waste products is believed by some physicians to relieve inflamed, congested kidneys of work and thus lessen further injury and give the kidneys a chance to recover from the damage already done" (Harmer & Henderson, 1939, p. 471). When I studied in Scandinavia, I learned that hot baths and saunas were recommended as a way to relieve the kidneys and allow the skin to act as a kidney for a short time.

Nurses used hot baths not only for stimulating excretion through the skin, but also to relax voluntary muscles, relieve pain, and to bring about circulatory changes in the skin and internal organs (Harmer & Henderson, 1939). Baths used for sedation were at skin temperature of 92°F. The bath was used for insomnia, comfort, and psychiatric conditions. A number of the retired nurses' narratives in Chapter 4 describe the historical use of baths for anxiety and nervousness. "A bath at body temperature produces no marked changes in the body, either thermic or circulatory, but surrounds it with a medium that shields it from all external stimuli, or irritation of nerve endings from air, clothing, pressure, changes in temperature, and the like. As a result, the nerve centers and whole nervous system are protected and allowed to rest. The bath is therefore soothing and quieting in its effects and gives a chance for repair and the storage of vital energy" (p. 475). It seems like common sense to use such a simple therapy. I have used sedative bath therapy with infants and found it helpful for relieving colic and improving sleep.

Packs are the wrapping of the whole body or parts of it such as the extremities in hot or cold sheets, dry or moist, and then wrapping the body up tightly. Today many nurses, physicians, and doctors of naturopathic medicine continue to use hot and cold packs for effecting change in a particular part of the body. Nurses still use ice packs to reduce swelling and hot packs, such as "hot pads," for back pain. The packs discussed in historical texts involve more than just applying hot or cold to the body. Like the art of bandaging, nurses learned the art of applying packs. Learning packs meant learning to *wrap* the body in some type of cloth or blanket as well as the application of hot or cold water. I learned to do cold and hot wraps for the feet following a footbath. It is truly an art that is best learned from a master.

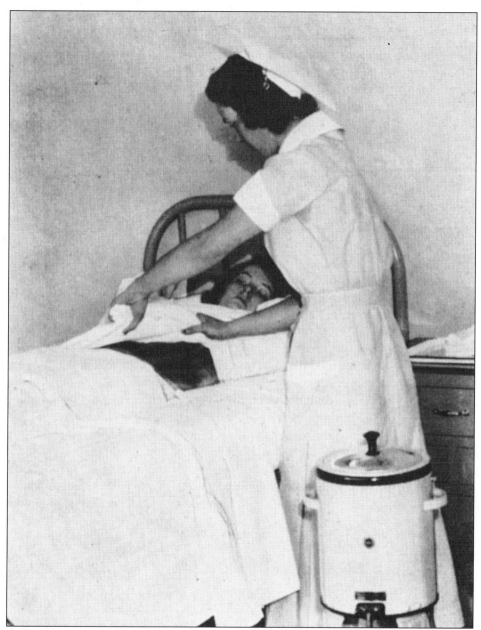

Hot stupes, also called hot packs, 1938 *(From Margaret Tracy,* Nursing: An Art and a Science. *St. Louis, MO: The C.V. Mosby Company, 1938. Used with permission.)*

Footbaths are still performed by some nurses. Bertha Harmer discussed the importance of the footbath. She writes, "The effects of this treatment [footbath] depend upon the temperature and the duration of the bath and upon the fact that the feet (and lower extremities) are reflexly associated with the brain, lungs, uterus, ovaries, bladder, and intestines. Any increase or decreases of the blood supply in the legs and feet will, therefore, have a marked influence upon the circulation of these organs" (1924, pp. 211–212). The purpose of the footbath has been to relieve "congestion" in the body. Moving the energy and blood in the body by giving a footbath was found to be helpful in conditions such as headache, nervousness and insomnia from overwork, sprained ankle, and gout; to relieve, prevent, or break up a cold or simple sore throat; to induce menstruation; to relieve pelvic congestion; and to stimulate the bladder or intestines.

Anthroposophical nurses use hot water bottles as part of a hot pack to deliver warmth. They believe that hot water bottles "communicate" warmth and nurturing to a patient and that heat produced by warmed water is steady, but gradually decreasing, which encourages the body to then heat itself. Elderly people love hot water bottles, especially for their feet. If applied to their feet, wrapped in a towel or flannel pillowcase so as not to be in direct contact with the skin, their feet can stay warm for hours.

Obstetric nurses are aware of the importance of hydrotherapies. They use hot tubs to assist the laboring mother, and sitz baths after delivery to encourage healing of the perineum. They also encourage fluid intake during pregnancy and lactation. All nurses learn the importance of bathing a patient. Not only is bath time an important time for hygiene, stimulating circulation, and comfort, but the bath time, as pointed out in many of the nurses' narratives in Chapter 4, is a time for the nurse to get to know the patient and talk with him. How a nurse gives a bath has also been very important. Elizabeth Gordon wrote in 1903, "Let the patient regard the process with pleasure, and not with dread. . . . Endeavor to be an artist in sponging. Know why you sponge. . . . Let your touch be gentle, firm and soothing" (Estabrooks, 1987, p. 38).

Conclusion

There is wealth of opportunity to promote the health and comfort of patients through the use of environment. Water, plants, air, sound, light, and temperature can all provide the foundation for simple yet profoundly effective caring modalities. Nurses can also participate in the creation of environments that humanize the health care experience of patients. Nurses have the ability to create healing environments with their patients that provide support for the processes of balance, understanding, growth, and achieving greater health and well-being. Nurses often underestimate the therapeutic value of their demonstrations of care through environmental modalities. Resources for further learning about environment and caring are provided in Appendix C.

References

American Association of Naturopathic Physicians. (1997). *A guide to alternative medicine.* Lincolnwood, IL: Publications International.

Bonn, D. (1998). Adverse drug reactions remain a major cause of death. *Lancet, 351,* 1183.

Brown, J., & Marcy, S. (1991). The use of botanicals for health purposes by members of a prepaid health plan. *Research in Nursing and Health, 14,* 339–350.

Capsaicin Study Group. (1991). Treatment of painful diabetic neuropathy with topical capsaicin: A multicenter, double-blind, vehicle-controlled study. *Archives of Internal Medicine, 151* (11), 2225–2229.

Cumming, J., & Cumming, E. (1962). *Ego & milieu.* New York: Prentice-Hall, Inc.

Davidson, A. W. (1988). *Choice patterns: A theory of the human-environment relationship.* Unpublished doctoral dissertation, University of Colorado, Denver.

Deal, C., Schnitzer, T. J., Lipstein, E., Seibold, J. R., Stevens, R. M., Levy, M. D., Albert, D., & Renold, F. (1991). Treatment of arthritis with topical capsaicin: A double-blind trial. *Clinical Therapeutics, 13* (3), 383–95.

Dehn, M. (1990). Vitamin C, chicken soup, and amulets: Students view self-care practices. *Nurse Educator, 15* (4), 12–15.

Enby, E. (1990). *Hidden killers: The revolutionary medical discoveries of Professor Guenther Enderlein,* S&G Communications.

Estabrooks, C. (1987). Touch in nursing practice: A historical perspective. *Journal of Nursing History, 2* (2), 33–49.

Farnsworth, N., Akerele, O., Bingel, A., Soejarto, D., & Guo, Z. (1985). Medicinal plants in therapy. *Bulletin of the World Health Organization, 63* (6), 965–981.

Green, M., & Keville, K. (1995). *Aromatherapy: A complete guide to the healing art.* Freedom, CA: The Crossing Press.

Grosart, D. (1995). Green matters. *Nursing Times, 91* (26), 48–50.

Haller, J. S. (1985). The poultice. *New York State Journal of Medicine, 85* (5) 207–209.

Harmer, B. (1924). *Text-book of the principles and practice of nursing.* New York: Macmillan Co.

Harmer, B., & Henderson, V. (1939). *Textbook of the priciples and practice of nursing* (4th ed.). New York: Macmillan Co.

Lawless, J. (1998). *Aromatherapy and the mind.* London: Thorsons.

Libster, M. (1999). Guidelines for selecting a medical herbalist for consultation and referral: Consulting a medical herbalist. *The Journal of Alternative and Complementary Medicine, 5* (5), 457–462.

McCarthy, G., & McCarty, D. (1992). Effect of topical capsaicin in the therapy of painful osteoarthritis of the hands. *Journal of Rheumatology, 19* (4), 604–607.

Moore, N., & Komras, H. (1993). *Patient-focused healing.* San Francisco: Jossey-Bass.

Negri, M.C., & Hinchman, R. (1996). Plants that remove contaminants from the environment. *Laboratory Medicine, 27* (1), 36–39.

Nightingale, F. (1957). *Notes on nursing.* Philadelphia: J.B. Lippincott Co.

Olson, S. (1998). Bedside musical care: Applications in pregnancy, childbirth, and neonatal care. *Journal of Obstetrics, Gynecology, & Neonatal Nursing, 27* (5), 569–575.

Parker, L. A. (1921). *Materia medica and therapeutics: A textbook for nurses.* Philadelphia: Lea and Febiger.

Pert, C. (1997). *Molecules of emotion: Why you feel the way you feel.* New York: Scribner.

Quinn, J. (1992). Holding sacred space: The nurse as healing environment. *Holistic Nursing Practice, 6* (4), 26–36.

Retallack, D. (1973). *The sound of music and plants.* Marina del Rey, CA: DeVorss & Co.

Robson, M., Heggers, J., & Hagstrom, W. (1982). Myth, magic, witchcraft or fact? Aloe vera revisited. *Journal of Burn Care and Rehabilitation, 3* (2), 157–163.

Roy, Sr. C., & Andrews, H. (1986). *Essentials of the Roy adaptation model.* Norwalk, CT: Appleton-Century- Crofts.

Smith, M. (1994). Beyond the threshold: Nursing practice in the next millennium. *Nursing Science Quarterly, 7* (1), 6–7.

Southwell, M., & Wistow, G. (1995). Sleep in the hospitals at night: Are the patient's needs being met? *Journal of Advanced Nursing, 21,* 1101–1109.

Tracy, M. (1938). *Nursing: An art and a science.* St. Louis, MO: C.V. Mosby Co.

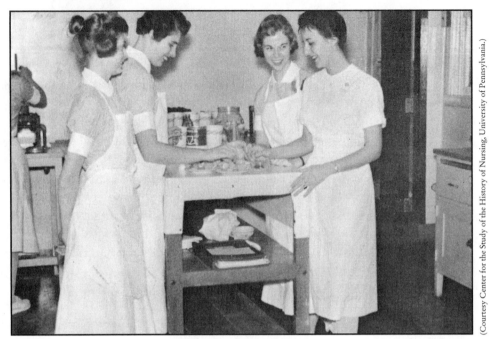

Nurses' cooking class

Food is an important part of a balanced diet.

—FRAN LEBOWITZ

CHAPTER 9

Nutrition: Nurturing with Food

The History of Food and Nutrition in Nursing Practice

The act or process of providing nutrition and nourishment has always been a basic element of the human experience. When one thinks of the act of nourishing, one often thinks of the mother feeding her infant. The infant needs food to sustain life but is unable to get the food or feed himself. The role of the mother is the bearer of life and health to the child. Nurses also have been seen historically as the bearers of life and health to the wounded and infirm, especially as they provide nourishment to patients. Although many nurses are involved with in-depth analyses of the patient's nutrition status and diet (e.g., with diabetic patients), this chapter concerns the more general and subtle aspects of demonstrating care by providing nourishment.

Nurses demonstrate caring by assessing the ability of a patient to take food and assimilate it. They attend to the various nutrition needs of the ill and convalescing as well as to patients who are well, such as babies, children, and pregnant women. Nurses provide diets to patients that modify caloric value, consistency, and food choice to meet the individual needs of patients. Florence Nightingale wrote of the importance of "punctuality" in presenting food to the patient and the nurse's need to use "observation, ingenuity and perseverance" when meeting the nutritional needs of the patient (Nightingale, 1957, p. 37). Many ill patients do indeed have specific times of the day when they are more capable of taking nourishment. Their readiness for food often depends upon their strength, emotional state, and the treatments they are receiving. When a patient is ready for food he should be positioned for comfort and nothing should distract him during mealtime.

Many historical nursing texts also discuss in great detail the arrangement of foods on the dish and the arrangement of the dishes on the tray to increase accessibility by the patient. Nurses have always been expected to feed patients who cannot feed themselves. "The enjoyment of a meal by a helpless patient who must be fed will depend largely on the nurse who feeds him" (Tracy, 1938, p. 102). Although nurses may understand the importance of nourishment to strengthening the patient's vital force, nurses often delegate feeding to assistants.

Yet mealtime provides an excellent opportunity for the nurse to assess many things about the patient's state of health. For instance, nurses can quickly recognize the patient's energy level and appetite while feeding the patient. In general, most nurses expect the digestion and assimilation of ill patients to be compromised. It has been the nurse's job to see to it that the patient has food that is easy to digest. "Since in many diseases diet is one of the most important therapeutic measures in the control of disease, and since all other therapies will fail if the patient is not properly nourished, the nurse should use every possible means to give the patient his correct diet, attractively and quickly served, while he is in the hospital, and, as far as possible, to insure continuance of proper dietary habits after he has been discharged" (Tracy, 1938, p. 102).

Florence Nightingale was very specific that the nurse's observation of the patient was key in determining the appropriate nourishment for the patient. She wrote, "Chemistry has as yet afforded little insight into the dieting of the sick. . . . In the great majority of cases, the stomach of the patient is guided by other principles of selection than merely the amount of carbon or nitrogen in the diet. No doubt, in this as in other things, nature has very definite rules for her guidance, but these rules can only be ascertained by the most careful observation at the bedside" (Nightingale, 1957, p. 42). Nightingale taught us the importance of the nurse's role in providing proper nourishment as that of first observing how foods are tolerated by the patient and then adapting the diet to facilitate "nature's" work. For example, the nurse who observes the patient during mealtime might notice extreme fatigue during or after the patient eats, indicating that the food may have been difficult for the patient to digest and assimilate. Nightingale considered diet and nourishment to be a "neglected" part of nursing work during her time. I would dare say that this may still be the same today.

COMFORT FOODS: DIET FOR THE SICK

As discussed in Chapter 6, the foods people choose when they are ill are often based upon cultural and childhood experiences. These are called *comfort foods*. Comfort foods vary according to time in history, person, and cultural beliefs. The patient's chosen comfort food often brings back a happy memory of a time when the patient felt nourished and cared for. When a patient eats a comfort food he tends to relax with a sense of satisfaction that goes beyond a feeling of fullness in the stomach.

Today's hospitalized patients are faced with diets ranging from Ensure, Jell-O, and ice cream to full steak dinners. These foods may or may not meet the patients' needs for comfort, let alone good nutrition. In the early 1900s, foods considered appropriate for the ill were foods such as beef-tea, beef broth, calves foot jelly, bran loaf, milk-punch, egg flip, oatmeal gruel, rice cream, wine jelly, tamarind whey, egg and sherry, mulled wine, peptonized food, and flour ball (Miller, Hunt, McCormick, Burr & King, 1914). I don't know if these foods were considered comforting to patients! Nightingale and other historical nursing writers provide explanation for the use of such foods. Specific dietary recommendations were made for many illnesses. The dietary recommendations were integrated with any other medical therapies prescribed. For example, there was a specific diet for the treatment of gonorrhea (Miller et al., 1914). Can nurses today explain how the foods they provide are assisting the patient's healing process? Is our role to just provide nutritionally appropriate foods? Is our role to just provide comfort foods? Perhaps part of the science and art of nursing is to be able to provide foods for patients that are both comforting *and* supportive of the healing process.

The Art and Science of Demonstrating Care by Providing Nourishment

The nurse's role in nutritional caring is twofold. First is that of provider of food and second is that of teacher. Nurses provide nourishment for those who cannot provide for themselves because food is necessary to sustain life. Food is secondary only to the air that we breathe and the water we drink. Nurses are the health team members who are usually responsible for the patient's nutritional status. Nurses also teach patients the science of nutrition and how to make appropriate dietary choices for themselves and their families. Nurses would probably agree with an ancient Chinese doctor named Sun Si-miao (who lived to be 101) that, "Those who are ignorant about food cannot survive" (Sun, 1993). Many nurses working in community health and with outpatients routinely teach their patients about nutrition.

Because of the tremendous variety in food choice and preparation among cultures, it is important that nurses perform a thorough assessment before making recommendations regarding any dietary practices. A person's dietary habits are often quite personal and nurses need to be aware that the food choices people make are not solely made based upon taste. They are made based upon psychosocial, sociocultural, developmental, and spiritual influences as well.

NUTRITIONAL ASSESSMENT IN NURSING CARE

One of the ways to demonstrate care regarding diet and nutrition is to assess the patient's need for nutritional assistance and/or education and his responses to the foods eaten. Table 9–1 is a sample of a nutritional needs assessment.

The observant, caring nurse, prior to giving any recommendations, takes the time to consider all of these factors. This holistic nutrition assessment is then followed by recommendations and patient education that is supportive of the ways in which the patient is already adequately caring for his own nutrition needs.

Keen nutritional observation and assessment, blended with a diplomatic approach to offering assistance, are important when dealing with peoples' nutritional habits and beliefs. For example, the importance of this holistic approach can be seen when working with mothers and their children, especially if the mother has been told by the physician that her children may not be growing well. It is a delicate situation to discuss diet and nutrition with mothers because they often feel personally attacked when someone questions whether their child is eating properly and/or growing. I have had numerous opportunities to discuss family nutrition status with mothers in

Table 9–1 Nutritional Needs Assessment

PHYSIOLOGICAL NEEDS

Nutrient/Caloric Requirements related to activity level that varies with age, sex, genetic, and metabolic processes as well as the integrity of body structure (Scheel Gavan, Hastings-Tolsma, & Troyan, 1988)

Appetite and thirst

Height and weight

Diet pattern

Food allergies

Condition of patient's mouth

Pain related to ingestion of foods or fluids

Sense of taste and smell

PSYCHO-SOCIAL NEEDS

Attitude, perception, feelings, and knowledge of nutrition

Social issues regarding food such as how food is prepared, what mealtime is like for patient, how often patient eats, and whether or not patient believes he/she has a socially and personally acceptable weight

Developmental changes that have affected dietary and nutritional habits such as preferences for certain textures and tastes and eating patterns related to age and development

SPIRITUAL NEEDS

Spiritual beliefs that influence food choices

my community health work. It was important to present any new nutritional information to the mother in a way that would not be perceived as threatening to her abilities to parent and nourish her children.

Often discussing *general* nutritional information with patients, such as the concept that "the body turns food into energy" or that "we are what we eat," opens the door for discussing the specifics of their nutritional choices. As the nurses' naratives in Chapter 4 identify, demonstrating care means not being judgmental of others. Patients need to feel that nurses do not judge their food choices and preferences and that nurses understand that everyone has a reason for eating certain foods at certain times.

Health care workers can never truly judge what food choices or meal patterns are "right" for someone else. Florence Nightingale showed us that nature and the individual patient will tell us this; but we can still learn more about foods and liquids and the physiology of digestion, so that when we talk with patients about diet we have a clearer understanding of their ability to digest and metabolize the foods they choose.

Consider eating seaweed, for example. I once worked with a dietitian who often recommended that her patients consider eating different types of seaweeds with their meals. Her explanation to patients was that the sea vegetables were "full of vitamins and minerals." As a nurse and clinical herbalist with the team, my job was to assess the ability of the patient to digest and metabolize the seaweed because most of the patients had never eaten seaweeds before.

Most of the patients said that they were not fully digesting the seaweed. I wondered, as they kept eating it, if they were truly getting their money's worth (seaweeds can be quite expensive). I went to a workshop on sea vegetation that was presented by a leading scientist in the field of algology, the study of algaes. It was fascinating to find out that what had happened to our patients happens to most people when they begin eating sea vegetables.

I learned that the body has to *adapt* to eating sea vegetables. Sea vegetables are clathritic, a term that means that the plant derives its nourishment from the passing seawater. When a human eats sea vegetables, the vegetable absorbs the body's fluids and minerals. The professor then described a program of introducing sea vegetables into the human diet without having adverse effects. One principle, he explained, was to eat the seaweeds as condiments in small amounts sprinkled on food and to significantly increase the amount of water in the diet. He explained that, over time, the body adapts to eating sea vegetables.

The ingestion of sea vegetables may sound completely unappetizing to some, but people of some cultures are used to a diet that includes small amounts of sea vegetables. For example, Japanese sushi is a little rice ball wrapped in nori, a type of sea vegetable. I use this example of knowing how to eat seaweeds as an example of the complexity of a single dietary recommendation or change. I have found that when addressing the nutrition needs of a patient, it is helpful to work closely with registered dietitians, patients, and their families. Nurses also work in collaboration with physicians providing observations and feedback on a patient's ability to follow a prescribed diet.

Patients also prescribe many different types of diets for themselves. One has only to go to the local bookstore to see the numerous diets that are recommended as the "key" to good health. Nurses cannot possibly be specialists in all of the physician and self-prescribed diets that exist. We can understand basic principles of nutrition, food preference, and human behavior. We do not have to understand the "chemistry" of every food, as Nightingale calls it, to be able to observe whether or not a food is appropriate for a patient. Patients often need assistance in choosing foods that they can tolerate based on the knowledge the nurse provides them on the nature of their illness and the potential benefits of any particular food. Although patients are ultimately responsible for what they eat, nurses are responsible for other important parts of nutritional caring, beginning with the presentation of the food to the patient.

FOOD PRESENTATION

Food presentation has been a part of the culinary arts for centuries. Presentation is the art of making a food or meal pleasing, appetizing, and digestible. "Awareness of presentation transforms a meal, helping one to eat less yet gain greater nourishment. . . . When accomplished as an art at the highest level, food presentation is elegant in its simplicity" (Pitchford, 1993, p. 231). Patients take in the way a meal is prepared and served as well as taking in the food itself.

Nurses have full understanding of the importance of the patient's ability to take in food and digest it. The patient's strength and vital power are dependent in part upon their ability to eat and digest. Historically, nurses presented and often prepared food for the patient. The understanding of food presentation entails understanding the timing of presentation, food portion, food color, and the way in which the food is offered to the patient. "Enjoying a meal depends on more than just the food that is consumed. The surroundings and how and when the food is served all influence the diner's feelings about a meal" (Sanford, 1987, p. 31). Why shouldn't patients enjoy a meal? Patients become quite uncomfortable when they have to eat a meal that is served at a time when they are not hungry, when the portion is too big, when the food is unattractive, such as being all one color, or when the tray is put before them without any thought regarding their ability to reach the food.

So often in hospitals the timing of a meal seems to be out of the nurse's control. The nurse does not serve the patient, and the patient often feels obligated to eat when they are served. Nurses can demonstrate caring by holding the meals for a later time and warming the food when the patient is ready for it. Patients should be told at the beginning of their hospitalization about this option so that they never feel pressured to eat. Patients need to be ready to digest their food. If they are upset or in pain they will not be able to eat as they normally do. Ideally, nurses would make sure that a patient is comfortable and ready to eat prior to receiving a meal.

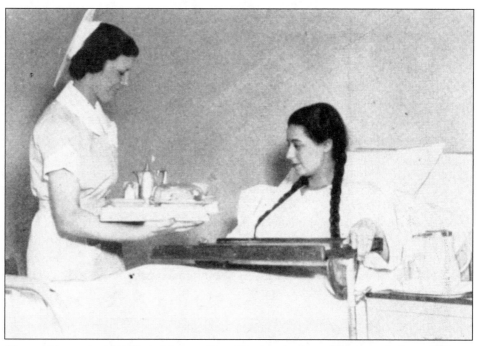

Dinner with a smile, 1938 *(From Margaret Tracy,* Nursing: An Art and a Science. *St. Louis, MO: The C.V. Mosby Company, 1938. Used with permission.)*

So often I hear of hospital patients complaining about the food. I have heard dietary service managers agonizing over how to improve the food. But history and present-day culinary arts show that the actual food is only one part of the issue. People know when the details of their meal are cared about. "At no time is one so particular about small things as when an invalid. This is especially so in regard to the articles of diet" (Miller et al., 1914, p. 154). This was written in 1914! People are particular about the little details such as whether the food is hot if it is supposed to be hot, if the food has color as well as taste, and if they are fed when they are hungry. In 1914 it was said to "give the patient his food very carefully—little at a time." How often are patients presented with a half a chicken? Even the small portions are too large for most ill people. More is not better. It takes energy for patients to chew and assimilate their food. Although they are supposed to get energy from food, some patients end up spending too much energy on chewing, either because they have dental problems or they are given a portion of food that requires too much energy to eat. This often happens with the elderly.

Chewing is important to digestion because digestion begins in the mouth. Many patients experience increased stress due to their illness and to a subsequent change of environment, such as being hospitalized. Their digestion is often affected. Patients need to be given time to chew and enjoy their meals and not feel rushed for any reason. They need to be given smaller portions and should be able to request more as needed. Nurses can demonstrate caring by attending to the needs of patients at mealtime.

COLOR.   Think of a meal you might have had where everything on the plate was one basic color: mashed potatoes, breast of chicken, wax beans and milk. Somehow it is not very appetizing. In the East, it is believed that food that is good for health should also be appealing to the senses. One important way to make food more appealing is to use color. It is believed that color attracts a person's qi or vital force. When our qi is attracted to food we want to eat it. In the East, a potato would not be served alone with chicken breast. Red or green pepper might be substituted or added for color.

In Asian medicine there is a belief that different colors have healing effects on different organs. One of the health theories in traditional Chinese medicine dating back to 400 BC, is called "five-element theory." In the five-element theory, a relationship is shown between the internal organs of the body and the seasons of the year,

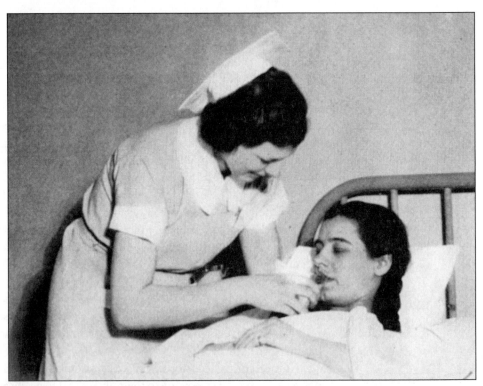

Sips of cool water, 1938 *(From Margaret Tracy,* Nursing: An Art and a Science. *St. Louis, MO: The C.V. Mosby Company, 1938. Used with permission.)*

colors, sounds, and other natural phenomena. "In five-element theory, the heart corresponds to red . . . the spleen to yellow . . . the lungs to white . . . the liver to green and the kidney to black. One should not memorize these lists of correspondences as dogma, but rather consider them as poetry, or a list of metaphors which may sometimes provide insights into observations or phenomena that might otherwise seem unrelated" (Rossbach & Yun, 1994, p. 113). It is believed that, in general, a person can eat certain color foods to affect the organ they wish to heal. Using color alone for healing any condition is never recommended but is included for general health purposes. There is an ancient science behind presenting the ill with a simple, yet colorful, meal.

DIGESTION AND EMOTION

A patient's ability to digest and assimilate food is affected by his emotional state. For example, a patient who is worried about the outcome of a medical test may have indigestion or loss of appetite. It is important to assess the patient for emotional reasons for change of appetite. It is also important to help the patient create an environment for the meal that is calm and supportive of digestion. Perhaps the patient would prefer not to eat alone and have visitors when eating. Every situation is different and the nurse demonstrates caring by assessing the social as well as nutritional needs of the patient at mealtime.

Love and caring are also important ingredients in food preparation and presentation. A friend of mine, Janice Feuer, who as a chef, has a talent for making food that is healing as well as tasty. She has written in her cookbook, *Fruit Sweet and Sugar Free,* that the four essential elements of fine baking are "love, technique, temperature, and recipe—in that order." The same is true in nursing and health care as with baking. The patient's food must be prepared with love and served with love and full reverence for the ability of the food to support the patient, the healing process, and the sustenance of the vital force. The techniques of the cooks and servers demonstrate how much they truly care about the patient's health. The food must be the right temperature. The love and effort behind the act of nourishing the patient is just as important, if not more important, than the food itself. Patients know the difference between food that has been prepared and served with care and that which has not.

One example of love and care in food preparation and service is the Japanese tea ceremony. The tea ceremony is a living art form in which the artist, by preparing tea for a guest, turns a "normal," daily event into a tranquilizing, beautiful ritual. "In the Tea Ceremony, the concern for beauty is so deeply pursued that tea can truly be referred to as an artform. Body movement is completely choreographed, even down to finger positions, and tea utensils can be of such high quality that you will find them in art museums throughout the world. . . . The rituals of the Tea Ceremony not only provide a patterned way of serving food and drink: they also demand that the

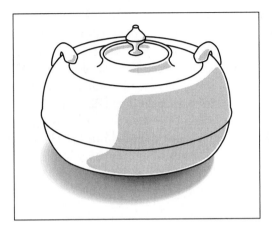

Japanese tea kettle

patterns have the dimension of beauty. . . . Taking care to see that food and drink are served beautifully tells the guests that the host considers them to be important people" (Keenan, 1996, pp. 31–35). The tea ceremony has been shown to have a healing (i.e., stress reduction) effect on both observer and performer as well. It is an ancient example of the establishment of a healing relationship through the art of nourishing another.

I wonder what patients would think if the level of attention taken with the tea ceremony were taken with their meal? I'm sure that there might be a patient or two who would say, "Why all the ceremony? Just put the pot on the stove and bring the tea as fast as you can." The question is, when it comes to healing, what's the rush? Rushing and stressing out is what makes many people ill. Is it possible that nurses could consider making the patient's food and nourishment, as well as its presentation, a nursing priority or even a ritual? After all, the best and most appropriate nourishment can be calming, satisfying, and healing. We are what we eat. We are how we eat.

Nutrition and Integrative Nursing

In an integrative nursing practice, the nurse creates healing relationships with patients by observing the patient's need for greater harmony and balance and then addresses those needs by offering care that is a holistic blend of biomedical and caring skills. The understanding of nourishment is integral to this practice. Food is vital to life and the proper food and nourishment are important to the quality of life.

As mentioned before, nurses do not define for patients what foods are proper for them, but nurses have an important role in helping the patient find the diet that they believe supports the patient's ability to have a long life. Most people want to live a long, happy life. The science of longevity is the study of what people do to help them live a long and healthy life. Many cultures have explored the concept of lifestyle practices, including diet, that affect longevity. Chinese emperors, for example, are renowned for their pursuit of the knowledge of longevity. They believed, as the Chinese people believe today, that diet is medicine. The traditional Chinese doctor prescribes no medicine or treatment until the patient's diet and lifestyle have been addressed. Often a change in diet and lifestyle is all that is needed to bring about the balance or adaptation that leads to the body's ability to heal with little or no further intervention. Nurses, like the Chinese, are often aware of the effects of certain foods on particular health conditions. For instance, the nurse knows by observation and education that a child who eats nothing but candy will soon become malnourished. Nurses have historically taught patients about nutrition and the principle of balance in taking all foods in moderation.

ALL THINGS IN MODERATION AND BALANCE

In the early 1990s, I studied traditional Chinese medicine (TCM). This course of study finally taught me the science behind the common sense of why foods should be taken in moderation. Because the Chinese use food as medicine, and many foods are plants, we learned the foundational theories of Chinese medicine and how they apply to food prior to studying the herbs used as medicine. We learned that foods have different taste, temperature, and energetic qualities. For example ice cream is cold, damp, and sweet, and chili peppers are hot, dry, and pungent. The science of TCM is based on theories of balancing the qualities, or symptoms and signs, exhibited by the patient, with the qualities of substances such as foods and herbs.

For instance, if someone has a cold and damp condition manifested by certain signs and symptoms, he would be given warm food to bring balance rather than a cold food, which would create greater imbalance. For thousands of years, the Chinese have perfected a health care system based on balance and common sense. The whole country has access to knowledge of this science much the way Americans had during the early 1900s with *Domestic Medical Practice,* the large set of guidelines provided for self-care. The Chinese, however, never gave up their traditional medicine. It is still alive today in hospitals in China. Many of the TCM concepts are complementary to Western nursing practice because of our understanding of the importance of promoting balance or adaptation within each individual.

Some basic principles in TCM diet therapy are congruent with nursing theory. For example, nurses know that the body's energy is derived from our food. The Chinese agree; they say that the qi, or vital power, is derived from the food that we eat. In order for this process to occur, the Chinese believe that foods must be eaten that support the warm digestive action of the stomach. The stomach is like a "pot on a stove." When the food is put in the "pot," it must be turned into 100 degree soup so that the "clear [part of the food] can rise and the turbid [the waste] can descend." There are many things that can affect the ability of the body to complete this process. That is what the student of TCM diet therapy studies. To give an example of the kinds of things taught in TCM philosophy and theory, imagine for a moment the digestive system as a pot on a stove that is trying to reach 100 degrees. What would happen if ice water were put into the pot? Of course, the pot would not have an easy time reaching 100 degrees. Someone would have to turn up the fire. TCM theory says that this is just what the body does to compensate. The extra fire can then cause something else to go out of balance and, although the Chinese know ways to ultimately create the balance, their philosophy is why put ice water into the pot in the first place? This is primary prevention.

The science of Chinese diet therapy involves the use of an "energetic" classification system of certain foods and herbs. The energetic quality of the food is hot, cold, or somewhere in between. In TCM, foods have a physical temperature in the range from hot to cold, and they have a postdigestive temperature also in the range from hot to cold. Postdigestive temperature refers to a particular food or drink's net effect on the body's thermostat. Some foods, even when cooked, are physiologically cool and tend to lower the body's temperature either systemically or in a certain organ or part.

In Chinese medicine, every food is categorized as either cold, cool, level (i.e., balanced or neutral), warm, or hot. Most foods are cool, level, or warm and, in general, we should eat mostly level and warm foods because our body is warm. "During the winter or in colder climes, it is important to eat warmer foods, but during the summer we can and should eat cooler foods. However, this mostly refers to the post-digestive temperature of a food. If one eats ice cream in the summer, the body at first is cooled by the ingestion of such a frozen food. However, its response is to increase the heat of digestion in order to deal with the cold insult. Inversely, it is common custom in tropical countries to eat hot foods since the body is provoked then to sweat as an attempt to cool itself down. In China, mung bean soup and tofu are eaten in the summer because both foods tend to cool a person down post-digestively" (Flaws, 1997, p. 15). In TCM, it is recommended that if a person must take ice cream or iced beverages, they should be taken between meals so as not to put out the fire needed for digesting a meal.

I have found in practice that there are many principles of TCM diet therapy that I can teach patients that appeal to their common sense. I find that by teaching these principles, such as understanding thermal quality of foods, I do not have to be in the position of "prescribing a diet." The patient then learns to choose his own foods, as he should. I do tell an ill patient not to eat the extreme foods, because it may take too much energy to restore balance.

The focus of nursing care is to help the patient preserve and enhance the vital force by helping him eat foods that sustain balance and harmony of spirit, mind, and body. Appropriate care related to nourishment helps to put the patient in the best condition possible for nature to assist him in healing. This particular modality of TCM was my choice to better demonstrate care by providing nourishment. It is by no means the only one, but has indeed been an important part of my development of an integrative nursing practice in which Western and Eastern nutrition science and the art of nourishment inform my nursing assessments and interventions.

WOUND CARE AND NUTRITION

One area of nursing care expertise that demands much attention to nutritional status of patients is wound care. A healthy nutritional status is essential to promoting wound healing. The goal of nutritional care for patients with wounds is to promote collagen synthesis. Some of the key nutrients for collagen synthesis are carbohydrates, protein, copper, iron, zinc, magnesium, and vitamins A, K, B_1, B_5, and C. Patients with wounds are in a catabolic state and, therefore, have an increase in dietary requirements. Catabolic means that they are in the second "phase of metabolism where complex nutrients are reconverted into more simple forms in order to release the energy necessary for cell function" (Hallett, 1995, p. 76).

Compromised nutritional status also predisposes a bedridden patient to pressure sores. This is especially problematic for the patient who, because of treatment (such as the cancer patient undergoing chemotherapy), has difficulty maintaining an adequate diet. Nurses play an important role on the health care team that provides nutritional care for patients with these specialized, often, complex issues.

EMOTIONAL WELL-BEING AND NUTRITION

In working as a school nurse, I often saw the impact of food on the emotional and psychological health of the students. Many students visited the nurse's office after having lunch in the cafeteria. It is also a well-known phenomenon among teachers and school nurses that many children are not very teachable after having sweets such as cake and ice cream at school birthday parties. The day after Halloween is a behavioral nightmare for most teachers. It is a common observation, and yet the research on the impact of simple sugar on children's behavior has not supported the hypothesis. There are many confounding variables in the research of how foods affect emotional well-being and behavior and much is still unknown. "A variety of dietary or nutritional treatment approaches have been reported to be effective for the alleviation of psychological symptoms. Clinical case reports suggest that a nutritionally unbalanced diet, vitamin and nutritional deficiencies, food sensitivities, intake of sugar and caffeine, and food additives and pesticides can have an effect on mental status. Yet the impact of diet on psychological health has not been widely recognized, extensively researched or incorporated into mainstream psychotherapeutic practice" (Miller, 1998, p. 54). I once worked in a group home with children with autism, developmental delays, and destructive behaviors. We observed and documented the impact of certain foods on the children's behavior patterns. There were indeed certain foods, such as beans and desserts, that seemed to be related to the children acting in a more destructive manner. These children demonstrated sensitivities to carbohydrate foods. Nurses are in a very good position to observe the impact of food on a patient's behavior and make modifications to promote well-being.

Conclusion

There are many ways nurses can be involved in the promotion of healthy dietary practices both in the community at large and in the biomedical world with its increasing complexity. Attending to nutritional needs of patients can provide that moment of beauty and simplicity of caring, such as with the Japanese tea ceremony, that patients *and* their caregivers need. The nutritional needs of patients cannot be left solely to the care of a dietitian and nursing assistant. Understanding nutrition needs, food presentation, and the impact of foods, diet, and the act of nourishing oneself on health and healing is vital to integrative nursing practice. Helping the patient to be nourished, body and soul, is a fundamental caring modality. Resources for further learning about nutrition are provided in Appendix D.

References

Flaws, B. (1997). *The tao of healthy eating: Dietary wisdom according to traditional Chinese medicine.* Boulder, CO: Blue Poppy Press.

Hallett, A. (1995). Vital ingredients. *Nursing Times, 91* (5), 76–77.

Keenan, B. J. (1996). The Japanese tea ceremony and stress management. *Holistic Nursing Practice, 10* (2), 30–37.

Miller, F., Hunt, H. L., McCormick, F. J. M., Burr, B., & King, M. (1914). *Domestic medical practice.* Chicago: Domestic Medical Society.

Miller, M. (1998). Diet and psychological health: A case study. *Alternative Therapies, 4* (2), 54–58.

Nightingale, F. (1957). *Notes on nursing.* Philadelphia.: J.B. Lippincott Co.

Pitchford, P. (1993). *Healing with whole foods.* Berkeley, CA: North Atlantic Books.

Rossbach, S., & Yun, L. (1994). *Living Color: Master Lin Yun's guide to feng shui and the art of color.* New York: Kodansha International.

Sanford, J. (1987). Making meals a pleasure. *Nursing Times, 83* (7), 31–32.

Scheel Gavan, C., Hastings-Tolsma, M., & Troyan, P. (1988). Explication of Neuman's model: A holistic systems approach to nutrition for health promotion in the life process. *Holistic Nursing Practice, 3* (1), 26–38.

Sun, J. (1993). Pillars of longevity. *Qigong, Health and Healing for the 21st Century* (Winter), 20.

Tracy, M. (1938). *Nursing: An art and a science.* St. Louis, MO: C.V. Mosby Co.

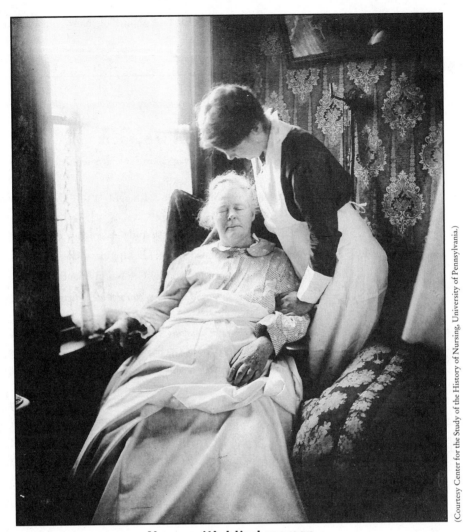

Nurse with blind woman

It takes two to speak the truth—One to speak, and another to hear.

—Henry David Thoreau

CHAPTER 10

Communication: The Healing Relationship

The History of Communication in Nursing Practice

The beauty and importance of many things are not felt alone; they are felt in relationship to something else. The blueness of the sky is only noticed because it meets the green and brown colors of the land. The height of the mountains is only noticed because of the valleys below. The night is noticed because of the absence of the sun. Yet so often we forget to absorb the vastness of the sky, or admire the strength of a mountain, or give thanks for the warmth and light of the sun because it all just *exists* around us and perhaps we take it a little for granted. Much about human relationships is the same. We know the similarities and differences between peoples. We wonder about how a relationship is born, how people come together like the sun meeting the darkness, or the mountain meeting the valley. Some relationships last a lifetime and others a very short time; but regardless of the time, relationships or interactions with some people are never forgotten. They touch our heart.

We make choices in life and some of the biggest choices we make are whom we want to have a relationship with; whom we want to be friends with, whom we want to marry, whom we want to do business with, whom we want to *care* for. Relationships always take two people. One person can start a relationship, but to be *in* a relationship requires two people and a connection. Caring relationships are no different. A connection is necessary for two people to have a caring relationship. Relationships can be seen throughout nature. We know the intimate relationship of the mother lion to her cubs, the bees to the queen bee, and the flock of geese as they rise in formation. Humans also need relationships, caring relationships. All relationships are founded upon the actions of the individuals who come together. Both people are equally important in the formation of the connection, even though, as in the case of the mother and her young, one in the relationship may be stronger and therefore take on the role of nurturer or caregiver.

Communication is necessary for the connection to occur in any relationship. Communication is the giving and receiving of thoughts, beliefs, and feelings. Throughout history, nurses have recognized the beauty and importance of communication with patients to build caring, healing relationships. Tracy says that, "The mechanics of nursing should never interfere with the establishment and maintenance of a relationship between the nurse and her patient which will enable her to help him to the fullest extent" (Tracy, 1938, p. 29).

The importance of the nurse's communication with a patient and his ability to create a healing relationship have been discussed in many nursing texts. Florence Nightingale discussed the verbal and nonverbal communication between the nurse and patient throughout her book, *Notes on Nursing* (1957). Tracy, Harmer, and Henderson discussed the nurse-patient relationship in their texts; and in 1952 Hildegarde Peplau wrote an entire book on the subject called *Interpersonal Relations in Nursing*. The importance of communication to the healing relationship is not new to nursing. Yet the literature shows, from Nightingale to the present day, the challenge is often for nurses to have the opportunity for necessary communication with patients to build a caring relationship. Nurses are often too busy with the "mechanics" or tasks involved in nursing care. "A study by Cosner (1965) showed that some nurses do spend time communicating with patients, but that the nurses who do communicate with patients tend to be students or nursing assistants, not the nurses in charge" (Fielding, 1987, p. 283). Most nurses value the opportunity to develop rapport with a patient and find a way to connect. However, it is sometimes a struggle to find the time to talk with and listen to a patient. Nurses are often overextended. In listening to the narratives of ten nurses in Chapter 4, I heard the same concerns from both the nurses who practiced years ago and from nurses presently in practice. It seems that nurses throughout history recognized the importance of communication with patients, yet finding the time to do it is an age-old concern. This chapter has been written with this concern in mind.

UNCERTAINTY DUE TO LACK OF COMMUNICATION

All patients, from the smallest child to the seniors of a community, are participants in their health care in some way. Because the role of the nurse is to facilitate the healing process, the patient is not dependent upon the nurse for healing but is often dependent upon the nurse for support, encouragement, education, and care. Nurses demonstrate care by providing a listening ear to the patient's concerns and by providing information and education based on the age, development, and the patient's ability and/or willingness to participate in his own health care. In order to do this, nurses use their skills of communication to meet the individual needs of the patient.

Patients are very different in their communication needs. In order for the relationship between the nurse and patient to be healing to the patient, the nurse observes the patient to determine how much interaction and what type of information the patient desires, as well as the appropriate moment to intervene. Some patients get extremely anxious if they know too much about the discussion of their doctors regarding the "possibilities" of diagnosis and/or prognosis. For example, a certain patient might feel more comfortable *not* knowing about test results. He might only want to hear the treatment recommendations from his physician. The nurse in attendance to this patient would know from the patient's behavior that he only wants to discuss treatment options.

Florence Nightingale describes the opposite situation where the patient *wants* to know about his condition and is kept in suspense so long that he suffers a "fatal response due to the uncertainty" (Nightingale, 1957, p. 26). To make matters worse, Nightingale reports that the doctor was seen by the fearful patient having a whispered conversation outside his doorway. Understanding how much the patient wants to discuss about his care and illness is a good example of one component of the complex dynamics of creating a healing relationship. It is important that the nurse find a way to connect with the patient so that the patient feels comfortable expressing his needs and concerns.

Patients often feel vulnerable from the insecurities of not knowing what to expect during an illness, from a change in lifestyle or environment, and from having to accept help from others, sometimes for very personal needs such as bathing. Nurses who develop a connection with a patient can use it as a point of reference for developing trust with a patient. The patient learns to trust that a complete stranger, the nurse, cares for him and that this nurse will come back when needed. As the patient develops trust in the nurse's ability to attend to his needs, his uncertainty and fear diminish and he is able to express himself more. Florence Nightingale uses the metaphor of light to explain the importance of developing a connection through supportive communication with a patient.

Nightingale writes about the importance of the nurse at the bedside. "When the sun is under a total eclipse or during his nightly absence, we light candles. But it would seem as if it did not occur to us that we must also supplement the person in charge of sick or of children, whether under an occasional eclipse or during a regular absence" (Nightingale, 1957, p. 23). The nurse is that "light" for the patient, a point of reference. She demonstrates this through communication with the patient. The nurse communicates both verbally and nonverbally that she is going to "be there" or "be present with" the patient to provide the care and support needed. The nurse earns the trust of the patient by demonstrating care through communication and by being *present* at the bedside.

PRESENCING

Many nurses, including the nurses in Chapter 4, associate the word *caring* with "being there" or "being present" for a patient. Nurses empathize with the feelings and experiences of the patient. Nurses talk with patients, listen to them, counsel them, and teach them. They hold patients' hands and offer a soft touch on the hand or shoulder to convey that they understand.

Nurses experience moments of connection with patients when, as described in the nurses naratives, the "monitors and IVs don't exist," everything in the room just "seems to disappear," and time stands still as they listen to the story the patient just has to tell. If you have ever had a connection with a patient, and had a moment such as this, you know that at that point in time, the caring modality was *you,* your ears, your thoughts, and your heart. You connect with the patient, human being to human being.

Patients often remember a nurse's *presence* with them more than any other treatment or experience during their illness. This is because the patient is aware that the nurse is able to enter *his* world, leaving the biomedical and nursing world for a moment, to explore what it means to *be* that patient. The nurse is able to "walk in the moccasins" of the patient, if even for a moment, to discover the meaning of the illness or concern the patient is dealing with at that particular moment in their life. As the nurse is present with a patient, he learns what the patient needs for balance and healing. Being *present* with a patient occurs when the nurse shifts her awareness from *doing* the caring modalities to *being* the caring modality.

One nursing study quotes surgical patients as saying that, "Attentive nurses make you comfortable" (Cohen, Hausner, & Johnson, 1994, p. 181). Patients in the study were very aware of the attitude of the nurse caring for them. They knew when a nurse was attentive or present with them and was able to meet their needs. Nurses are present with patients in many ways. Sometimes nurses are present by being the emotional support for the patients when they are experiencing fear about their health. Sometimes nurses are present by making sure that patients have everything they need, such as a clean room, fluffed pillows, and a snack at the bedside. Sometimes nurses are present by offering words of encouragement to a laboring mother. Sometimes nurses are present by sitting down with a patient and asking them how they feel, and then waiting for the full story after the patient says the usual "fine." Nurses who are present with a patient are attentive and responsive to patient needs in the moment. It is the ability of the nurse to be in the present moment that supports the patient's ability to change and adapt. The future and the past cannot be changed. Nurses help patients find meaning in the past. They help patients explore future possibilities. But the patient and nurse can only effect change in the present moment. Nurses are the health care providers that interact with patients moment to moment. It is easy to see why *presencing* in nursing practice is so common. Although the therapeutic "value" of a nurse's presence is only beginning to be studied, nurses need no research or justification to be present with patients. Having a nurse as the "light" or presence at the bedside of the patient is just the humane and compassionate thing to do.

The Art and Science of Demonstrating Care by Communicating with Patients

Although some nurses seem to have an innate gift for communicating with patients, effective communication is a skill that is acquired over time. Nurses learn how to communicate effectively with patients by watching other nurses, taking classes in communication techniques, and from their patients. Communication is a science *and* an art.

THERAPEUTIC USE OF SELF

In addition to the nurse being with the patient, the patient must *be* with himself to participate in the healing process. Nurses use interpersonal communication skills that allow for the emergence of the *being* of the patient. The nursing intervention of being present for a patient, and of providing the environment and opportunity for the patient to explore himself, is called the therapeutic use of self. Nurse theorist, Lydia Hall, called the therapeutic use of self, the "core" of the nursing process. She wrote in 1964 that, "It is impossible to nurse any more of a person than that person allows us to see. In the process of exploring with a nurse—who he is, where he is, where he wants to go and will he take or refuse help in getting there—the patient will make rapid progress toward recovery and rehabilitation. . . . The nurse who uses herself therapeutically, must not allow her own concerns to interfere with the patient's exploration of *his* concerns. Besides this, her learning experiences through the media of the social sciences must facilitate the development of interpersonal skills that permit the patient to *be* and in being, to participate in facing, solving and preventing health problems" (p. 152).

Patients need guidance during the healing process. They need someone at the bedside, a point of reference, to help them as they find out what participation in a healing process is like. They need support in finding their own way through the process, in their own time. When acting as guides, nurses use themselves as an instrument of healing. They enter into a relationship with the patient, based on the needs and desires of the patient to enable the patient to learn about himself, body, mind, and spirit. The experience is never the same for the patient or the nurse because people, with all their basic similarities, are so very different. Each healing relationship is different.

For example, I had a very heartwarming experience with a patient when I was providing phone counseling, a nursing activity in which therapeutic use of self, in particular the voice, is the caring modality. The patient called to discuss the upper endoscopy she was to have the next day. She said that she was calling to discuss the benefits and risks of the procedure; but, when she said that she had called before for the same information, I knew that there was something else she needed in addition to information. As we started talking about the benefits and risks of endoscopy, she began to discuss her anxiety about the procedure. She had had the procedure before and was found to have an esophagus that was half paralyzed. The other half of her esophagus was functioning normally.

As we talked more about her anxiety and fear about the procedure, which was being done for diagnostic purposes, she talked about her doubts that the second endoscopy would give her any new information. She said that she knew that she might go through a lot of discomfort for "nothing." I heard a lot of fear, doubt, and anxiety, three common emotions patients express to nurses when they begin to trust.

This patient thought that there was a possibility that her doctors "really didn't know what was going on." I could tell that she wanted to be a very active participant in her care and so I asked her what *she* thought was "going on" with her esophagus. Her initial response was, "I don't know," so I asked her to close her eyes and think about her feelings about the endoscopy and the paralysis of her esophagus. I asked her to do something a little strange. I asked her to ask her esophagus what was wrong. I told her that every part of her body has intelligence and wisdom just as she, as a whole person, has intelligence and wisdom.

I learned this "body's inner wisdom" technique from my work in dance and from reading a book by a physician named Dr. Christiane Northrup, *Women's Bodies Women's Wisdom* (1998, p. 53). I had used it many times and found it to be a helpful and often enlightening experience for patients. This woman said she would like to try it so she closed her eyes. There was a period of silence on the phone for about thirty seconds and then I heard her say, "Ohhhhh!" I asked her if she would like to share what she was told. She said that she had been "told" that the cause of her paralysis had a lot to do with her feelings about her multihandicapped daughter.

She had a twelve-year-old daughter from a previous marriage who was completely dependent upon her. She and her present husband also had a four-year-old daughter. Her present husband was very accepting of the older daughter and yet the woman felt so "guilty" that she, her husband, and the four-year-old had never really been able to "bond" as a family because of the incredible needs of the handicapped daughter. The woman said that she and her husband had been talking about putting their older daughter in a foster home for a while so that they could spend more time with the younger daughter. The woman said, "Half of me wants to put her in a foster home and half of me does not. . . . Half of me can *swallow* the idea and the other half of me cannot *swallow* the idea." That was her "ah-ha" moment. She said that in order to be well she was going to have to work on the guilt feelings and make a decision either way. I just listened to this exceptional woman come to a profound realization. What a precious moment it is to *witness* the inner wisdom of another human being.

Such a simple communication technique and yet so profound an example of the importance of developing the therapeutic use of self. I don't know what the outcome was for this patient, and I probably will never know, but I know that it was a healing moment for both of us. We experienced the power of the healing relationship and I experienced the importance of communication as a means of achieving connection.

Communication with patients and getting to know them as the unique people that they are is energizing for many nurses. It is also good for the health of patients. "There is now considerable research evidence to demonstrate that good communication practices actually assist the rate of patient recovery and decrease reported pain, drug usage, postoperative complications, and length of stay: in short, they are cost effective" (Fielding, 1987, p. 282).

LISTENING FROM THE HEART

Hildegarde Peplau writes, "Observation precedes interpretation of the collected data. If giving advice is to be used as a technique in counseling, careful observation and skillful listening always precede the giving of advice. When nurses develop and use a technique of listening that is largely non-directive and non-moralizing the patient will gradually discover facets about himself that he did not recognize before; a series of such discoveries in the course of any illness may for some patients prove illuminating and therapeutic" (1952, p. 69). When nurses listen with the intent of being a sounding board and a point of reference, the patient is then free to express himself without trying to please. He can *be* himself.

Nurses who listen often hear the patient's hidden emotions, thoughts, and beliefs. It is important for the patient to be able to feel comfortable to talk about whatever they feel is important. No nurse can force a patient to discuss his thoughts or feelings. Patients who sense the support of the nurse will reveal what is in their hearts. A nurse who is listening with her heart will be prepared for the patient who wants to talk heart-to-heart.

Listening with the heart is an important part of "active" listening. Often nurses are told to be active listeners and how to respond while a person is talking. Nurses are never told how to deal with the thoughts that come to them while listening, thoughts that can affect their ability to be completely present and listen. In order to fully *hear* what the patient is saying, the nurse must listen with the heart, not just the ears. Listening from the heart means being completely focused on the three elements of the patient's communication. These three elements of heart listening have been defined by Sara Paddison as the *words*—what the patient actually says; the *feelings*—the feelings behind the words; and the *essence*—the real meaning (1995, p. 203). To listen from the heart is an active, compassionate caring modality. It takes the ability to put one's own thoughts on hold as they come up, and they do. Heart listening also means that the nurse puts all advice on hold until the patient is finished speaking and the nurse has identified the essence of what has been said.

Waiting for the patient to finish is important because the essence of what the patient is saying may not be revealed at first. The patient will feel "heard" if the nurse is able to respond not only to his words but also to his feelings and the essence or hidden meaning of what he is trying to say. Oftentimes, patients don't actually verbalize their feelings or the essence of what they are experiencing. Many times they express these things in nonverbal ways. Peplau writes, "In nursing it is necessary to find out more than the patient tells directly. Indirect communication occurs through words and through actions that can be de-symbolized and their hidden meaning identified or at least speculated on. . . . Nurses can ask themselves, in most situations, what the patient is saying through his complaints about his bodily functioning, about personnel, about his family. *What is the patient saying that he cannot say in any other way?"* (1952, p. 295). When a nurse takes this investigational approach to heart listening, it is difficult to hold onto judgments and opinions that, although part of the human experience, can interfere with the development of a healing relationship with a patient.

It is human nature to form judgments of others. Nurses who are able to deeply listen to patients are those who learn through experience how to put those judgments aside and meet the patient where he is. Sara Paddison writes, "There will always be people with whom you feel more resonance than others. There will also be people with whom you don't feel any resonance at all. You can still love them without judgement. Tune into their essence. That's one of the serious practices of self-empowerment—to be in the heart and love people, whether or not there's a resonance. Practice sending love and care whenever irritations or judgements come up. . . . You just build tolerance and compassion for every type of person you meet" (1995, p. 115).

Nursing is a profession that offers ample opportunity to build tolerance and compassion for others. It is not always easy because patients who are scared and sick are not always the most loving and compassionate people. Communication and relationship building in nursing practice can be challenging and energizing or it can cause great turmoil and stress.

Communication is a modality that has always been part of nursing practice. Every nurse knows that when she *knows* a patient a little better it is easier to care for that person; it takes less time because the nurse can then anticipate the patient's needs. It takes time and energy on the part of the nurse to communicate with a patient.

ENERGIZED TALK

Because communication and the healing relationship involve both the nurse and the patient, the nurse also has communication needs. Just as the patient needs to be supported and empowered by communication with the nurse, the nurse needs to be empowered by communication with patients. One way nurses can feel empowered is by communicating a positive image of themselves and their practice when they speak with patients.

The words we choose to communicate reflect our thought processes. For instance, when a patient asks for something and the nurse, unable to fulfill the request, says very politely, "I'm sorry but I can't do that for you now" the patient only hears the words "I can't." Patients don't like to hear these words; no one does. The patient may become angry with the nurse and communication and trust can break down. If a nurse knows the request cannot be granted, but says to the patient what she *can* do first, the patient is given a very different image or impression. The patient hears, "I can do it, but maybe at a different time" (a time that will fit with the nurse's busy schedule). This practice of telling a patient what can be done, meeting both the patient's and nurse's needs, can be energizing. Saying "I can't" all day long can be taxing to one's self-image over time. Because nurses are continually busy, and working with needy people, it becomes important to know ways to communicate to meet the needs of patients and ourselves. Energizing talk is one way.

I have used this communication technique a number of times and have found that my whole outlook on my work changes. I feel a greater sense of empowerment. For example, a patient asked me to get her to the shower immediately. I knew that I

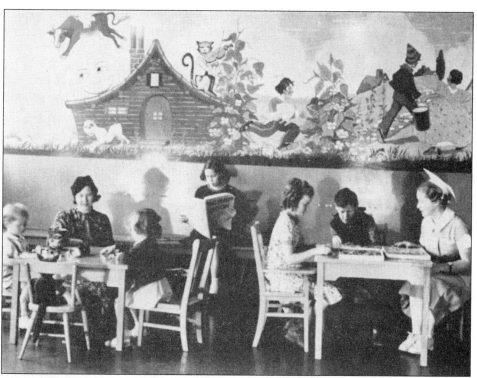

Nurse with children in waiting room, 1938 (*From Margaret Tracy,* Nursing: An Art and a Science. *St. Louis, MO: The C.V. Mosby Company, 1938. Used with permission.*)

had to help a doctor with a procedure, so I told the woman what I *could* do. I told her that I could help her in fifteen minutes after I assisted a doctor, or I could have the nursing assistant help her now. I never said that I couldn't help her now, but I definitely communicated that message. As if by magic, patients seem to be much more accepting and understanding when you don't say the word no one wants to hear—no.

Another energizing communication technique is speaking decisively. Have you ever asked someone to help you with something, only to be told that they will do it "when they get a chance," that "they will try," or that they "might get it done" at a certain time? This can be unnerving. It is not easy to trust that the help is forthcoming. Patients experience the same feelings when caregivers are indecisive. They depend upon a nurse to help them with the most intimate details of their daily existence and are told, "When I get a chance" or "I'll *try* to do it." Not very reassuring! In fact, it often is quite anxiety-producing. Nurses can avoid having to spend the time dealing with a patient's anxiety and fear by being proactive and saying exactly when they will meet the need of the patient. "I will help you at eleven o'clock if that will work for you." Nurses can also be proactive and discuss a patient's needs at the beginning of a shift if in a hospital or home care situation. For example, the nurse can find out ahead of time what the patient's expectations are and let the patient know early on when she will be checking in. Checking in is one way to develop trust with patients who often ring their call lights out of insecurity and loneliness.

TIME TO COMMUNICATE

Being a nurse-communicator is important in the health care environment, yet nurses often perceive that there is "not enough time" to communicate with patients. In all the historical texts on nursing practice that I have read, I never once found a book, journal, or newspaper article that said that nurses have "all the time they need" to do the caring work expected of them, including talking with patients. Throughout history, some of the perceived obstacles to having the time to talk with patients have been things such as having too many patients during the war, health care organizations' devaluing the importance of bedside nursing, and managed care. There has always been some external source of pressure that challenged nurses' abilities to develop a relationship with their patients. Because the pressure doesn't seem to go away, the question then is how can nurses continue to have the time to communicate with patients and provide an opportunity for the healing relationship to emerge? This question needs to be addressed because communication with patients is foundational to nursing care.

Communication is what many nurses do so well and what the patient often remembers most about his health care experience. Nurses can take more responsibility in their organizations for creating a nursing environment that is able to support the value of the healing relationship between nurses and patients. Nurses can also, on an individual basis, create a dialog with patients that expresses their desire to spend time with the patient while acknowledging the limitations of the situation. Sometimes nurses need to say to patients, "I wish I could spend more time with you right now but I'm going to have to come back later." The nurse must be able to observe the communication and interaction needs of patients so that she can be present at the right time, for each patient.

Nurses know when they are not providing for the communication and support needs of patients. If given the choice, nurses can create staffing models that take into account the needs of the patient for "time with a nurse." Historically, this time for communication happened during the back rub or the daily care the nurses performed. Now that the nurses in many health care facilities spend less time performing daily care, the patients may never talk with a nurse. What happens to nurses when they are no longer *present* with patients? What happens to nurses when the foundation of the healing relationship—communication—breaks down or is nonexistent? Do patients go elsewhere to get their needs met?

Communication and Integrative Nursing

Communication and the healing relationship are foundational to integrative nursing practice. Without communication, nurses cannot adequately assess the need for an intervention, whether biomedical or caring. Without communication and a relationship with the patient, the nurse cannot be a resource for the patient to achieve greater balance with his environment. Communication and healing relationships emerge as the nurse, through observation and intervention, addresses each unique patient's need to express himself.

When patients are diseased or uncomfortable, they often have strong emotions. They have many questions and concerns and they wonder to whom they can turn for help. Patients turn to nurses for help because the role of the nurse has always been defined in society as "one who will care." Caring is the foundation of the nurse-patient relationship. In the practice of integrative nursing, caring can be expressed through the modality of communication. The goal is to understand the patient. Greater understanding of the patient enables the nurse to interact with a patient in a holistic way that is appropriate, timely, and meaningful. The three concepts that form the basis for understanding and communication in integrative nursing practice are empathy-sympathy-respect, instilling hope, and mindfulness.

EMPATHY, SYMPATHY, RESPECT

Hildegarde Peplau introduced the concept of empathy, taken from the field of psychotherapy, into nursing literature in the 1950s. Prior to that time the word *sympathy* had been used. Florence Nightingale said that the nurse should be "kind and sympathetic." "By the 1930's, there was an increasing awareness of the psychological aspects of patient care (Tracy, 1938); sympathy was reinstated in nursing as an 'essential' quality (Harmer and Henderson, 1939) that enhanced the nurse-patient relationship and the therapeutic process" (Orlando, 1961; Peplau, 1952; Morse et al., 1992). Empathy has been described by Morse as both a feeling and a therapeutic modality or response used in patient care. Empathy and sympathy are just two of the many responses nurses have when relating with patients. Respect is another feeling and therapeutic response that is often present between nurses and patients.

There is no question that a nurse should be respectful of her patients, but the "appropriateness" of other feelings and therapeutic responses such as sympathy and empathy are not as clear. *Should* a nurse be sympathetic or empathetic? Some nurses are taught to be empathetic and some sympathetic.

I remember being taught as a nursing student that sympathy was not appropriate but that empathy was. Nurses are aware of having emotions toward patients and being confused about what is an "appropriate" feeling. In Chapter 4, Joan discusses being reprimanded for being "unprofessional" because she cried with a family when their child died. Was she being sympathetic or empathetic or both? Was Joan right in crying with her patient's family? Her head nurse said no. After years of practice and experience Joan still believed that what she did was not wrong. She still believed in her decision to cry with the family at that time. Nurses decide every time they enter a relationship with a patient just how emotionally involved they will be. It's not always a decision that comes from the nurse's head. Some nurses decide with their hearts. Joan's was a decision of the heart.

Perhaps our heads tell us that it would be convenient if there were a rule about how much interaction and emotional involvement to have with a patient. Having spoken to retired nurses who practiced under this type of rule years ago, I learned that there was still ambiguity and concern about how emotionally involved to be with patients. Nurses struggled with the question of professional distance then just as nurses do now. Is it really something we need to answer for our profession as a whole? Or can it be something that nurses are taught to attend to as part of developing a healing relationship with a patient? Can one nurse tell another nurse how much emotional involvement to have with a patient? Is that even possible? It somehow seems impossible for one nurse to tell another how to feel about a patient. How a nurse acts on those feelings, i.e., with sympathy or empathy, may be a different situation. How nurses act on their emotions is a way of demonstrating care that is very personal and unique to the individual nurse. Because healing relationships are so unique and circumstantial, it would be controversial to suggest that there is a right way and a wrong way of demonstrating emotion in a professional relationship.

Dinah Gould, in her discussion of the professional status of nursing, raises the issue of "sieving through only those likely to fit the mould" (Gould, 1990, p. 1171). By nurses learning that one therapeutic response is favorable to another are we not asking nurses to "fit a mould"? "If learners (nursing students) are progressively encouraged to abandon their own individuality, they are unlikely to value this quality in patients through empathic understanding" (p. 1171).

Nurses need to understand the full range of emotions they will experience personally with patients. This type of learning is often experienced in a relationship with a mentor, someone the nurse can trust to share emotions with. Nurses who receive this type of emotional mentoring and support in school and in practice are often better able to deal with the complex emotional issues that come up in developing healing relationships.

Nurses who are more comfortable in the process of exploring their own feelings will also be better equipped to understand and validate this process with patients. Nurses demonstrate care for a patient when they respond to the patient in a way that validates their feelings. Peplau gives a good example of a nurse who negates the patient's fear of dying in the hospital when she responds to the patient by saying, "Oh, but you aren't going to die, we will take care of you." Peplau says, "This remark, in effect, denies the validity of the patient's feelings and in order to feel safe the patient may have to give up attending to what he feels and indicate verbal acceptance of what the nurse has indicated he *should* feel. . . . Nondirective listening offers the patient a sounding board against which he can reveal feelings and discover them" (1952, p. 29). Validating a patient's feelings is a clear way to demonstrate caring, empathy, sympathy, and respect.

Another way to demonstrate caring, respect, and empathy, through nonverbal means, is by going physically to the patient. Home health and public health nurses do this all the time. One nurse educator found the laundromat to be an ideal place not only "suitable for the wellness end of the health continuum and for promoting health and preventing illness" but also for the instruction of nursing students in initiating interpersonal relationships (Eggebroten, 1973, p. 762). Pediatric nurses kneel down when providing care to their young patients. Taking the caring to the patient, where he feels comfortable, builds trust with community members. Trust, acceptance, and the healing relationship are earned over time. They provide the framework for the health care provided in a community.

INSTILLING HOPE

In the high-tech, biomedical world so full of the newest understanding of medicine, diagnostics, and treatments, there is often great hope offered to those who suffer; hope that they will soon be free of their suffering. The thought of a cure brings hope to patients. It is not only the thought of cure that can instill hope. Patients experience hope from their caring relationship with nurses as well. Communicating or instilling hope is one part of being present with a patient. One study with cancer patients identified the need of patients and their caregivers for nurses and doctors not to give up and to "be there and remain hopeful" (Ferrell, Zichi Cohen, Rhiner, & Rozak, 1991, p. 1317).

Nurses must remain hopeful so that they can help patients feel hopeful. Margaret Tracy has described instilling hope as part of the nurse's knowledge of "mental hygiene." She quotes Mary Beard (1936) as saying, "There is in nursing a power to create in the patient so strong a desire to live that it may become the one factor which decides the issue in the patient's struggle with disease. And it is not only in the individual patient struggling with the issues of life and death that nurses may plant this vital seed, but in a family, in a neighborhood; in the falling infant death rate of a state or a nation, the creative power of good nursing is vividly manifest to one who looks for it. I am inclined to believe that unless a nurse has this conception of the possibilities of constructive change in the patient's attitude of mind, she cannot do real nursing" (Tracy, 1938, p. 32). Nurses must be able to hold a vision of the patient as having all that is needed to heal. Reason for hope exists in every situation.

Instilling hope does not mean that nurses disregard or, as Nightingale says, "make light of danger." She discusses in detail the difference between true hopes and the "chattering hopes and advices" that are often given to patients. "I would appeal most seriously to all friends, visitors and attendants of the sick to leave off this practice of attempting to 'cheer' the sick by making light of their danger and by exaggerating their probabilities of recovery" (Nightingale, 1957, p. 55). Nightingale says that patients given this kind of chattering hope are found wanting of sympathy. " He feels what a convenience it would be if there were any single person to whom he could speak simply and openly, without pulling the string upon himself of this shower-bath of silly hopes and encouragements; to whom he could express his wishes and directions. . . . An infant laid upon the sick bed will do the sick person, thus suffering, more good than all your logic. A piece of good news will do the same" (pp. 57–58). Nurses need to find ways to instill hope and inspiration in patients, not only through words, but also by actions that bring life to and around the patient. Instilling hope means involving the patient in life, even if his own death is part of that life.

MINDFULNESS

Knowing how to interact with a patient, how to be with a patient, how to communicate with a patient, how to respond emotionally to a patient, and how to instill hope with patients requires the nurse to be conscious and aware of what is going on with the patient, herself, and the environment. Each moment with the patient can be experienced by the nurse who has entered the world of the patient. Moment to moment awareness has been called "mindfulness." Jon Kabat-Zinn, who uses the concept of mindfulness in helping patients in his stress reduction and relaxation program at the University of Massachusetts Medical Center, describes the concept of mindfulness as a "way of paying attention . . . the complete owning of each moment of your experience, good, bad, or ugly. . . . Cultivating mindfulness can lead to the discovery of deep realms of relaxation, calmness and insight within yourself" (Kabat-Zinn, 1990, pp. 11–12). Kabat-Zinn's patients are taught mindfulness living practices such as meditation. The program has been very successful in helping people with physical problems that are aggravated by stress.

Mindfulness is not a new concept for nurses. Since Florence Nightingale and probably before, nurses have valued the importance their own state of mindfulness, referred to as calmness, keen observation, or the ability to focus, and of helping patients to maintain a calm, relaxed state as a means to accessing their inner strength for healing and health. Nurses exhibit mindfulness in their use of communication, presencing, counseling, relaxation, and guided imagery techniques to help patients.

Historically, nurses have talked of relaxation as "providing comfort," both physical and mental comfort. Nurses were taught hydrotherapies and massage as modalities to be used to encourage patients' relaxation. The effects of relaxation have to do with the "deep rest brought on by focused attention on a simple mental stimulus such as a word, phrase or image. This focused attention is associated with decreased sympathetic nervous system activity, resulting in lower heart rate, blood pressure, respiratory rate, metabolic rate, and muscle tension . . . the opposite of the stress response" (Wells-Federman, 1996, p. 20). Mindfulness practice is a way of eliciting the relaxation response, for example, focusing attention on breathing. Nurses use this relaxation technique with people in pain, such as women in labor.

Another mindfulness practice is to engage every sense in the experience of eating. Look at the food, smell the food, taste the food. Focusing on the smallest experience such as eating an orange, can be very relaxing. Patients who are hospitalized often have very little they can do to relieve their stress, so engaging them in relaxation and mindfulness exercises can be helpful.

I once took care of a six-year-old girl who was very worried about the medicine going into her IV. She was scared at the thought of the medicine reaching her body and not knowing what it would feel like. We talked about it. I explained the purpose of the medicine and that her parents agreed with her doctor that the medicine would be helpful for her. I also told her that I hoped there was something we could do so she would not be afraid of the medicine going into her vein. I asked her what her medicine would look like if it were a helping medicine. She said that she visualized the medicine as her favorite color, purple. I asked her to close her eyes and use her mind to "see" the beautiful purple medicine helping her body. She lay back on her bed and closed her eyes as I started the IV medicine. Soon she was able to open her eyes, see the medicine going in, and not be afraid. She always called that medicine her "beautiful purple medicine." Imagery and other relaxation techniques such as this can be quite helpful in quieting a patient's fear response. Many patients have their own relaxation techniques they use for coping with difficult situations. Nurses can be supportive and caring by asking patients about their ways of relaxing before engaging the patient in a stressful treatment situation.

Conclusion

Communicating with patients can be a vital, energizing part of nursing work that includes the dynamic exchange of thoughts, beliefs, feelings, hopes, support, and care between two unique individuals. Communication, both verbal and nonverbal, is a way of demonstrating care and is foundational to the development of an evolving, healing relationship. Resources for further learning about communication are provided in Appendix E.

References

Cohen, M., Hausner, J., & Johnson, M. (1994). Knowledge and presence: Accountability as described by nurses and surgical patients. *Journal of Professional Nursing, 10* (3), 177–185.

Eggebroten, E. (1973). Why not the laundromat? *Nursing Outlook, 21* (12), 758–762.

Ferrell, B., Zichi Cohen, M., Rhiner, M., & Rozak, A. (1991). Pain as a metaphor for illness. *Oncology Nursing Forum, 18* (8), 1315–1321.

Fielding, R. G. (1987). Communication training in nursing may damage your health and enthusiasm: Some warnings. *Journal of Advanced Nursing, 12,* 281–290.

Gould, D. (1990). Empathy: A review of the literature with suggestions for an alternative research strategy. *Journal of Advanced Nursing, 15,* 1167–1174.

Hall, L. (1964). Nursing—What is it? *The Canadian Nurse, 60* (2), 150–153.

Harmer, B. & Henderson, V. (1939). *Textbook of the principles and practice of nursing* (4th ed.). New York: Macmillan Co.

Kabat-Zinn, J. (1990). *Full catastrophe living.* New York: Dell Publishers.

Morse, J., Anderson, G., Bottorff, J., Yonge, O., O'Brien, B., Solberg, S., & McIlveen, K. (1992). Exploring empathy: A conceptual fit for nursing practice? *IMAGE, 24* (4), 273–280.

Nightingale, F. (1957). *Notes on nursing.* Philadelphia, PA: J.B. Lippincott Co.

Northrup, C. (1998). *Women's bodies, women's wisdom.* New York: Bantam Books.

Paddison, S. (1995). *The hidden power of the heart: Achieving balance and fulfillment in a stressful world.* Boulder Creek, CA: Planetary Publications.

Peplau, H. (1952). *Interpersonal relations in nursing.* New York: G.P. Putnam's Sons.

Tracy, M. (1938). *Nursing: An art and a science.* St. Louis, MO: C.V. Mosby Co.

Wells-Federman, C. (1996). Awakening the nurse healer within. *Holistic Nursing Practice, 10* (2), 13–29.

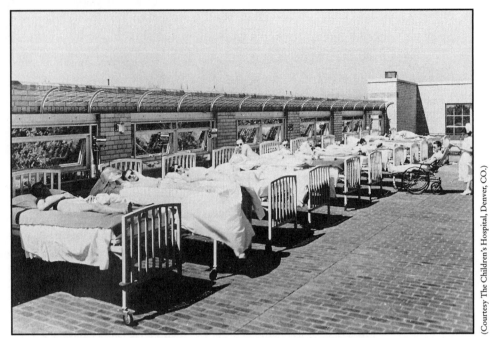

Nurse supervising heliotherapy

Better to light a candle than to curse the darkness.

—CHINESE PROVERB

CHAPTER 11

Energy Therapy: Understanding the Body Energetic and Magnetic

The History of Energy Modalities in Nursing Practice

Throughout history, nurses have helped patients conserve energy, preserve energy, build up their energy, and restore energy. Often "energy" has been called "strength." Nurses perform duties that help preserve the "strength" of the patient. Florence Nightingale called the patient's energy or strength the "vital power" (Nightingale, 1957, p. 9). Nurses, at least since the time of Nightingale, if not throughout the history of nursing, have been concerned with the preservation of the patient's energy, or vital power, so that he might use his energy for healing. All work, including the work of healing, requires energy. The body's innate tendency is to restore balance at the cellular, organ, and system levels. This balancing process that occurs in the patient's body and between the patient and his environment is critical for adaptation and survival. This process takes energy. Anytime the nurse attends to the patient's ability to preserve and enhance balance and life, and to heal, the nurse works with the patient's "energy."

Chapters 7–10 discussed the nursing fundamental modalities of touch, the environment within and without, nutrition, and communication. All these modalities, in fact all nursing tasks and patient responses, involve the use of energy. Energy is life. Energy is motion. If the heart stops beating, there is no motion; there is no life. If the body does not move, disease can easily take over. If a person's thoughts don't move, thoughts, such as "I am a failure" or "I'm going to kill someone," the person can become ill, mentally and often physically. If a person's spirit doesn't "move," and he becomes stuck in a sense of hopelessness or lack of power, he can become ill. The movement of energy in spirit, mind, and body is essential to health and well-being. The concept of the nurse's role in preserving and strengthening the vital power is prevalent throughout Nightingale's book on nursing practice. The concept of energy, and a human being as an energy field is also prevalent in the writings of more recent nurse theorists, such as Martha Rogers, Rosemarie Parse, Margaret Newman, and Jean Watson. The concept of energy is foundational to both nursing and to all modalities used in nursing practice whether they are biomedical or caring skills. This chapter discusses the concept of healing energy or vital power in its many forms.

All civilizations have been conscious of the energetic and/or magnetic forces influencing human life. Earlier civilizations explained illness as the work of external forces of the spirit world. "Certainly, by the advent of written history, medicine had already evolved into a complex belief system centering on the life force and body energies. Treatments for influencing these energies involved magic, herbs, and natural forces of magnetism and electricity. By all criteria, the system we call 'primitive' was not only well developed and sophisticated, but was actually a kind of energy medicine" (Becker, 1990, p. 12).

The Chinese system of health care incorporates the concept of energy as qi (pronounced chee). It is believed that the movement of qi throughout the body, in pathways called meridians, is essential to life and that the blockage of qi can lead to imbalance and disease. Chinese healers, after thousands of years, continue to successfully affect the health of the Chinese people with the use of modalities that move or unblock qi, modalities such as herbal medicines, acupuncture (the placement of needles into the skin along the meridians), and moxibustion (the use of heat on points along a particular meridian). The Chinese, early Egyptians, Indians, and Tibetans used the magnetic properties of the lodestone for healing as well.

In addition to vital power, Florence Nightingale spoke of the energy the person gleaned from warmth, fresh air, and light and the importance of these to the healing process. She knew the healing art and science of opening the windows to freshen the air of a sickroom while preserving the temperature of the room. She knew that a "careful nurse" was one who guarded against the patient's loss of "vital heat." Nightingale refers to both "vital" heat and "vital" power. Vital refers to vitality, or having to do with life. The preservation of warmth and energy are fundamental to nursing care.

Nurses are also aware of the importance of light to the healing process. Tracy discusses the importance of sunlight in patient care. "The proper lighting of a room is important to the mental and physical comfort of the patient as well as to his safety. Sunlight, which has a marked germicidal power, is therefore an important disinfectant. Man has found by experience that sunlight is desirable in human dwellings and an effective aid to healthy living. The placing of the bed where the patient can enjoy the effects of the sunshine without the discomfort of having the light directly in his face is one of the nurse's responsibilities" (Tracy, 1938, p. 37).

Nightingale discusses the importance of sunlight. She compares humans and plants in that each face the sun or turn toward the sun. "It is direct sunlight they want. . . . People think the effect is upon the spirits only. This is by no means the case. The sun is not only the painter but the sculptor. . . . Light has real and tangible effects upon the human body. . . . Who has not observed the purifying effect of light, and especially direct sunlight, upon the air of a room? The cheerfulness of a room, the usefulness of light in treating disease is all-important" (Nightingale, 1957, p. 48).

The historical American nursing texts of the late 1800s and early 1900s specifically discuss the modality called *ray therapy* or *heliotherapy* as the use of the sun in nurses' healing practice. In the United States, Colorado has had many clinics specializing in the use of the sun bath, or heliotherapy, to heal many types of "tuberculoses," such as lung, ribs, larynx, genitourinary tract, and intestines. Sunbaths were also used for persistent pneumonias. Doctors prescribed change in climate for their patients and sent them to clinics in sunny places with dry air, such as Colorado Springs and Glenwood Springs, Colorado. "In the sun, the temperature is warm and equitable; it is never cold, and during midwinter, and in fact during the entire winter, invalids sit on the piazzas of their houses in the open air without extra wraps. The thermometer when exposed to the sun's rays indicates from 90 to 130 degrees of heat, and there is always a difference of at least 50 degrees between the sun and the shade" (Knight, Wagner, & Chateris, 1889, p. 8).

The nurse heliotherapist was expert in the field of "ray therapy." Ray therapy included both the use of sunlight and the use of incandescent light. In ray therapy, the nurse knew how much radiant energy to apply to the body. The light bath was used for conditions such as "relieving internal congestion and pain" by increasing the volume of blood in the skin, to promote the absorption of "inflammatory products," to promote the formation of new tissue in the treatment of wounds, as a "tonic" to the skin and tissues, and to elevate body temperature quickly. "The vitalizing and healing power of the sun's rays has been recognized and utilized in the treatment of the sick from the most ancient times. They not only stimulate the circulation and all the activities of the skin, but penetrate to the inner most parts of the body, vitalizing, restoring and promoting the vital activities of every tissue" (Harmer, 1924, p. 367).

Nightingale also knew the importance of the sunlight to both the spirit and the mind. "One of the greatest observers of human things (not physiological), says, in another language, 'Where there is sun there is thought.' Put the pale withering plant and human being into the sun, and, if not too far gone, each will recover health and spirit" (Nightingale, 1957, p. 49). Recent research has confirmed Nightingale's belief in the effect of light, or lack of light, on the human spirit. Light has been shown to be an effective antidepressant treatment for seasonal affective disorder (SAD) (Terman, Terman, & Ross, 1998). "But light is as effective as drugs, perhaps more so. . . . Light is now recommended as the treatment of choice for SAD. . . . In addition to SAD, new applications for light have recently been summarized in the Society for Light Treatment and Biological Rhythms Task Force commissioned by the American Sleep

Disorders Association: for circadian-related sleep disorders, aging and Alzheimer's disease, jet lag, and shift work" (Wirz-Justice, 1998, p. 861).

There is no doubt that energy, in the form of light, has historically been associated with health of spirit, mind, and body. For many years nurses have observed the beneficial effects of sunlight and other light sources to human life. Nurses created and continue to utilize light therapy modalities in practice, such as placing babies in the sun or the use of ultraviolet light in assisting the baby's body to conjugate bilirubin. "Ott's (1973, 1985) research suggested that full-spectrum light may be essential to human well-being. His extensive work over more than twenty years implicated the use of frequency blocking devices, such as sunglasses and sunshields, with many health problems including arthritis and cancer" (Davidson, 1988, p. 59). The use of energy and light in healing is nothing new to nurses. There really isn't anything "new under the sun."

The Art and Science of Demonstrating Care with Energy

The more one learns about the human body, the more one realizes that there is so much more to explore and learn. As nurses, we witness in our patients the miraculous force of energy at work in the body demonstrated in the processes of restoration, recreation, and rejuvenation. We watch bones heal and people survive severe trauma. We witness the delicate "thread" of life working in the lives of patients and we know how quickly that thread can be severed. These experiences generate a respect and a desire for greater understanding for the complexity of the inner workings of the human body.

Some nurses dedicate their lives and careers to understanding the care of patients with a particular diseased organ. I have a colleague who works in an eye surgery center and is an expert in the care of patients with debilitating eye conditions. The eye is fascinating. It is an organ of tremendous ability in that the cells of the eye regenerate very quickly. One could spend a whole lifetime just studying the eye. The nurse who works with patients with serious eye conditions, helps patients *see* themselves, their families, their world, and their illnesses, and gain meaning from their experience of sight, or lack of sight, as well as helps them deal with the physical symptoms of eye disease.

Nurses who specialize in working with one organ or one disease process can still practice holistically. Nurses care for the whole person, a being that is complex and truly miraculous in structure, function, and spirit. They take into account each and every aspect of the life in their care. Nurses care for a life, that regardless of age, is powerful, energetic, and replete of potential. The nurse's role is often one of assisting patients in accessing their inner potential, their inner energy for healing. This potential exists in the vital power of the patient. The nurse who cares for patients receiving eye surgery witnesses the vital power in the regeneration of the eye. Florence Nightingale knew this as she created an environment for nature to work with the patient. Nurses today learn more about the potential of the vital power of the patient as research provides greater understanding of the developing science and art of the *use* of energy in nursing practice.

Nurses who work in radiology understand the use of energy such as X ray, computed tomography (CT) scan, and magnetic resonance imaging (MRI) in the diagnostic process. Surgical nurses have experienced the use of energy in the treatment of the surgical patient with laser and cauterization. Medical nurses use heat lamps to promote wound healing and provide chemical drugs and intravenous solutions that create huge chemical and energetic changes in the body of a patient. Numerous modalities used in nursing that harness energy, either the body's innate energy potential or energy sources from the environment, can create an effect on the body's energy field both within and without.

The body is energy. All matter is energy. Albert Einstein demonstrated this in his theory of relativity, $E=mc^2$, in which energy is put equal to mass multiplied by the square of the velocity of light. Mass can be converted into energy and vice versa. Therefore the nurse must assess the *energy,* or vital power, of the patient before, during, and after all interventions. The three areas involved in the art and science of demonstrating care with energy are understanding *energy* itself, the *movement* of energy, and the *flow* of energy.

ENERGY, MOVEMENT, AND FLOW

Energy exists in many forms. Energy implies the capacity of the body to do work. As in the examples of the way nurses use energy in practice, it can be seen that energy exists in forms such as heat, electrical energy, chemical energy, gravitational energy, magnetic energy, and energy of motion. Energy always implies action. Energy can be transformed, but can never be lost. One of the most fundamental laws in physics is the law of conservation of energy: no energy can be lost. Therefore, based on this law of physics, the body, as a mass or a form of energy cannot be lost. It can only be transformed into another form of energy.

All forms of energy can also affect the body. We have seen this in the practice of medicine especially with the use of chemical drugs. It is not only the chemical energetics of the drugs that affect the body. "Recent developments in quantum physics have led some scientists to suggest that electromagnetic energy in medicines interact with the body on some level" (Friedman, Sedler, Myers, & Benson, 1997, p. 955). I was once told a story about nuns who used their hands to bless the medications they gave to patients. The way I remember the story is that the nuns prayed over the medications they gave so that there would be no side effects to the medications taken by the patients. They were very successful. Did the electromagnetic energy of their hands in some way affect the electromagnetic energy of the drug and its impact on the patient?

The Chinese have recognized the electromagnetic energetic as well as the chemical energetic qualities of drugs for some time. The Chinese classify herbal medicines as well as Western pharmaceutical medicines not only by their chemical constituents and actions on the body. The medicinal substances are also classified for their energetic qualities, for instance whether they are warming or cooling to the body or whether they move energy (qi) or blood.

Eastern and Western healing modalities all address the importance of moving energy. You may have heard someone say, "I need to get my blood moving . . . my circulation isn't very good. I need to get myself up out of bed . . . or I feel constipated." These are all examples of discomfort due to a lack of motion or blockage of the flow of energy. "According to Chinese medicine, areas of energy flow blockage result from imbalances (disharmonies), which eventually are manifest in the form of disease" (Olson, 1998, p. 570).

Pain in a particular muscle is a good example of the blockage of flow. When a muscle becomes tight and the blood vessels of the muscle become constricted, there is decreased blood flow to the area, a diminished oxygen supply to the muscle, resulting in pain, one of the body's protective mechanisms to call attention to the area. Patients have many choices as to how they can deal with the pain. They can use chemical energy, i.e., a drug to override the pain response. They can use their strength or energy to mentally block out the pain response, an action often seen as "doing nothing for the pain," when in fact tremendous energy is required to block out the pain response. They can also use their mind's energy to create a relaxation response in the muscle, allowing the blood, and hence the energy, to flow again through the muscle. Then the patient would need to identify why their muscle tightened up in the first place so that the blockage does not occur again. Pain can recur if the signal is suppressed or ignored. It can even get louder.

"The key to treating such recurring conditions of disease may not lie in simple, 'quick-fix' physical solutions, but in the realm of re-patterning the organizing energy fields which direct the cellular expression of dysfunction" (Gerber, 1988, p. 44). This repatterning is enhanced by the careful observation and caring intervention of a nurse who understands that the "Band-Aid" will eventually come off and that healing involves more than the resolution of symptoms. Healing involves learning from the experience. Taking the muscle pain example again, the nurse who dispenses the muscle relaxant or the pain medication is only partially helping the patient understand the reasons for the pain. The nurse is in the perfect position to help a patient understand the body's response to tension as well as the effect of the mind and emotions on the stress response the patient experiences. The nurse can also utilize multiple modalities that address the holistic needs of the patient, as opposed to just easing the pain with a pharmaceutical intervention.

Nurses observe various energy levels in patients, energy flow, and energy blockages. Every cell, organ, body system, the body as a whole, and the person herself experience the flow of energy and the potential for blockage of energy and disease.

The nurse is also aware of the tremendous potential for energy to influence the healing of the patient. Nurses are constantly removing barriers and blockages to the flow of energy experienced by the patient. A very simple example is assisting the patient to get out of bed and sit up in a chair. How simple and yet how profound an experience for someone who has not sat up for days. We help the patient gain the strength to sit up and when the time is right, we provide support and encouragement for the patient to get out of bed because we know that it improves circulation as well as the spirit.

Flow implies movement. Take the flow of breath. There is a movement of air into the lungs, movement of oxygen and carbon dioxide in or out of cells throughout the body, and movement of carbon dioxide out of the lungs. We do not think about inspiration, respiration, or expiration, but it happens. Think about the beating of a heart. All four chambers move rhythmically and powerfully every day, all day. We do not think about it, but it happens. Energy is movement. Energy is all around us. Although we are not always consciously aware of the energy around us and in us, it does not mean that it is not there.

I remember consciously experiencing the energy around my body for the first time when I was standing on a stage during a rehearsal for a dance performance. I had never noticed it before, but when the lights were turned on me, especially the lights from below so often used in dance production, I could trace energy patterns in the air with my body. I could see the energy radiating out from my body because of the right lighting. I learned that my body was energy and light, and that it *interacted* with light. I can only imagine what the first scientist to x-ray the human body felt like when the first picture was viewed, or what the first surgeon to open the chest thought when he actually saw the heart. Sometimes it takes years before science has the ability to observe and measure certain human phenomena. As we move forward in nursing, we can only wonder at the things we will learn about the vital power and how we, as nurses, influence it knowingly and unknowingly in ourselves and others, either for good or for ill.

RHYTHM, FREQUENCY, AND VIBRATION

Rhythm, frequency, and vibration are also important to the understanding of energy. Rhythm is defined as, "A movement or fluctuation marked by the regular recurrence or natural flow of related elements." Frequency is defined as "the number of repetitions of a periodic process in a unit of time; the number of complete oscillations per second of energy in the form of waves." Vibration is defined as, "Oscillation; a rapid to-and-fro motion of the particles of an elastic body or medium that produces sound; a characteristic emanation that infuses or vitalizes someone or something and that can be instinctively sensed" (Merriam-Webster's Collegiate Dictionary, 1999). All three words denote energy that regularly occurs and can be heard and/or sensed in some way. All life is energy, rhythm, frequency, and vibration. Patients' bodies have rhythm, frequency, and vibration. Nurses do, too. Each individual patient and nurse has a unique vibration. That vibration or frequency changes during interaction with the environment and changes in thought and emotion. Human beings are in constant motion and undergo constant frequency changes.

Integrative nurses, who understand the importance of energy in practice, must be continually aware that their thoughts, emotions, and behaviors not only contribute to the environment of the patient, but contribute also to the changes in the energy field around the patient. The patient's energy also contributes to the changes in the energy field of the nurse. Whenever we come in contact with a patient there is some kind of energy exchange. Conscious awareness of this process enables the nurse and patient to demonstrate greater reverence for the relationship as the means to accessing a tremendous vital power of both the nurse and patient. The energy-conscious nurse observes the changes in a patient's frequency and vibration, manifested in their emotions and thoughts brought on by certain interventions that affect mind and body. The concept of mind-body medicine is not as new as some might think. Florence Nightingale wrote, "Volumes are now written and spoken upon the effect of the mind upon the body" (Nightingale, 1957, p. 34). Scientists and healers throughout the ages have understood the importance of the flow of energy in the body and the energetic connection between mind and body. Energy, in its many forms, affects the whole person.

Nightingale speaks to the power of energy for mind-body healing in her examples of flowers and light. She says, "I shall never forget the rapture of fever patients over a bunch of bright-colored flowers. People say the effect is only on the mind. It is no such thing. The effect is on the body too. Little as we know about the way in which we are affected by form, by color, and light, we do know this, that they have an actual physical effect. Variety of form and brilliancy of color in the objects presented to patients are actual means of recovery" (Nightingale, 1957, p. 34). Nightingale knew, as do many nurses today, that the energy involved in our caring interventions with patients, whether it's a touch, a flower, or other change in the environment, can have a powerful healing effect.

HARMONY AND ORDER

There is tremendous healing energy and potential in the simple tasks that nurses do every day with patients. The nurse performing these seemingly mundane tasks of cleaning off a bedside stand, straightening the covers on a bed, and throwing out trash can be dismissed as inconsequential. In a fast-paced health care environment these tasks can often be completely overlooked with the greater goal of "getting people well" with treatments, surgeries, and high-powered drugs. What difference does it make if the patient's room is cluttered?

Is there any value in cleanliness and orderliness to the health of the patient? To babies there seems to be a difference. I have found that the babies whose cribs were clean, with straightened sheets and a limited number of play objects in the crib actually sleep longer and deeper than the ones whose cribs are disorganized.

Harmony and order are energy terms. Harmony and order imply vibration or frequency, a wave pattern that is pleasing. The terms *harmony* and *harmonious* can be used to refer to music, color scheme, and relationships. "All uses of harmony convey a sense of unity and equality of form, a comfortable patterning. Predictable harmony in environmental wave patterns has been related to rest in human beings. . . . The harmonious flow of energy between human beings and environment has also been related to human well-being. Grad (1967) found evidence of greater health and well being among plants and animals that received water handled by happy persons versus depressed persons. Grad considered that energy had been transmitted to the recipients from the energy field of the giver. Higher energy in the giver was related to improved well-being in the recipient" (Davidson, 1988, p. 50). Harmony as a type of energy-based caring modality can be healing.

Nurses often deal with people who are suffering, not feeling a high level of energy, and may not be very harmonious. If the energy of a high-level giver (the nurse) can be transmitted to a lower-energy recipient (a patient), how does a nurse maintain her high level of energy? Nurses can become drained of the energy needed to be harmonious in providing patient care. When this happens, nurses cannot help anymore; they become tired. Nurses need to care for themselves by recognizing when their energy "tank" is empty. Nurses need time to reenergize in their own way. Some nurses reenergize with sleep; others need more than sleep.

Nursing is a practice of giving of the self, of one's *energy,* time, and resources to others. The question of providing a source of energy to patients cannot be taken lightly. The more nurses give, the more they need to be conscious of the flow and exchange of energy and what the energy exchange feels like with different types of patients. Nurses can identify whether one patient needs more energy than another. Embracing the differences in patients, the differences in relationships with patients, and the differences in the energy shared with patients helps caregivers adapt, remain flexible, and ultimately flow *with* the stream of energy involved in caring for patients rather than across or against the stream of energy. Flowing *with* the stream promotes harmony and the possibility of entrainment with the patient.

ENTRAINMENT

In the 1600's, Dutch scientist Christian Huygens, first noted a scientific phenomenon known as entrainment. Huygens found that one source of rhythmic vibration can cause another to vibrate *in sync* with the first. A common example of the occurrence of entrainment is a cuckoo clock shop. Eventually a time comes when all the clocks' pendulums swing in complete synchrony with one another. Other common examples of entrainment are the synchrony of the menstrual cycles of a group of female coworkers and the synchronization of a newborn baby's respiratory rate with its mother's.

Also the heart rate variability (HRV) of an individual who is calm and in a happy state of mind shows entrainment of the sympathetic and parasympathetic nervous systems. Researchers who study entrainment at the Institute of Heart Math have found that when a smooth HRV rhythm is created by a person with pleasant thoughts, "when head and heart, thoughts and feelings are working together harmoniously, the person feels greater balance and clarity and feels better" (Childre, 1994, p. 41). We entrain within ourselves and with others and our environment. A mother and child have the potential to entrain, or gain synchrony with each other. People entrain with their pets. Because all life is movement, vibration, and rhythm, there is potential to entrain and experience oneness and harmony with all life.

Often, people who practice some form of meditation describe a feeling of peace with themselves, as well as a feeling of oneness with their environment, even the universe. As scientists look closely at these experiences, some interesting correlations are made. "It is interesting to note that deep space, the earth's magnetic field, and brain wave activity of persons in a meditative state (low/alpha/theta) all vibrate at approximately 7.8 Hz per second" (Williams, 1993, as qtd. in Olsen, 1998, p. 570). Perhaps the feeling of oneness can be explained by the energy experience.

Applying the knowledge of the possibility of entrainment can lead to greater understanding and empathy with patients in health care environments. Greater under-

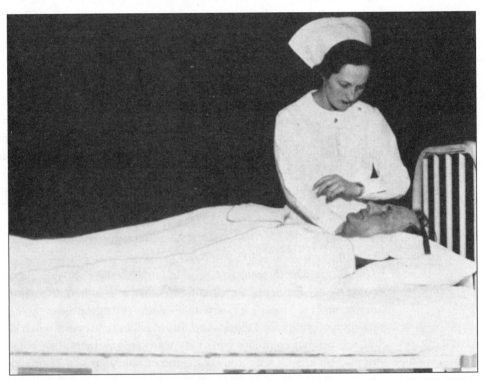

Pyrotherapy, 1938 (*From Margaret Tracy,* Nursing: An Art and a Science. *St. Louis, MO: The C.V. Mosby Company, 1938. Used with permission.*)

standing can lead to less effort and energy needed to work with the patient. An example of when less energy is needed to work with a patient is in continuity of care in a hospital or community health center. Often it takes much longer to perform basic nursing duties the first day of taking care of a patient because the nurse doesn't know the patient or his preferences. Getting to know the patient takes energy and effort. After the nurse gets to know the patient and his routines, the medication and treatment schedule, comfort needs, etc., she no longer has to ask the patient what he needs; she intuits and anticipates his needs better with each subsequent day of care.

I have found this to be especially true with nonverbal clients such as small children and infants. Once I know the mother and baby's schedule and rhythm, it is so much easier to take care of them. Observing the subtleties of the use of energy in demonstrating care can lead to greater comfort for nurses caring for patients as well as the patients themselves. There is much to be explored in the science and art of the use of energy in nursing practice. One can only imagine the profound impact a greater understanding of energy fields, vibration, color, and light can have on the ability of a nurse to demonstrate care.

Energy and Integrative Nursing

History has shown the use of energy in nursing practice. From heliotherapy to radiology, nurses have been specialists in the use of energy in health care practice for decades. Recently, more nurses have become interested in the subtle use of energy for promoting healing and health. Nurses have been involved in exploring the science and art of using music, guided imagery, and movement in nursing practice. Nurses use music for comforting hospitalized children and infants, teach stretching and yoga for cardiac rehabilitation patients, and provide guided imagery and visualization opportunities for cancer patients.

The use of energy is not really new to nursing practice, although some of these modalities may seem new. Picture a nurse from long ago holding an infant in her arms, singing a lullaby (music therapy) to the baby to coax it to sleep. Picture nurses from long ago before there were physical therapists working in hospitals. These nurses exercised, massaged, and danced with their patients to encourage movement. Picture wartime nurses at the bedside of a wounded soldier listening to his stories of home as he uses memory and visualization to recreate a happier time in his mind in an attempt to deal with the horrors of war. Nurses know all about music, movement, and visualization. It is only more recently that many of these modalities have been formally introduced to the public as separate specialized healing modalities.

MUSIC

Music has the potential to soothe body, mind, and soul. Rhythms, cords, harmonies, and melodies can stimulate memory, cause distraction from unpleasant circumstances, generate an emotional response, and uplift the spirit. Music has the potential to heal. The choice of music for healing is very personal. Not all people feel uplifted by a Puccini aria. Not all people are energized by the music of the Rolling Stones. Taste in music has a lot to do with life experience, culture, and vibration. Just as two people may feel greatly attracted to each other, a person and his music are attracted to each other. One man's music may be another man's noise.

The nurse who chooses to use music for healing begins by providing music that is individualized for a particular patient. "Bedside musical care involves more than just the bedside playing of music chosen by a patient. It involves the larger phenomenal process of creating a spiritual space with the patient. . . . Music holistically affects the healing process, even when cure is not possible. . . . Bedside musical care by its very nature involves validation of the patient and the moment. . . . Bedside musical care uses the phenomenon of entrainment and the qualities of tone, rhythm, pitch, and volume to affect the healing process" (Olson, 1998, p. 571). Nurses who use music as a therapeutic modality often are able to *connect* with patients in a way they are not able to when trying to communicate verbally. "Creation of meaning of a musical selection is in the mind and imagination of the person. Is this not the process of creating significant form to one's human condition? It becomes a way of creating connectedness among, at times, apparently fragmented and broken discontinuities. The aesthetic, sense-filled experience of music making and/or music listening may create a connection across the gap" (Chinn & Watson, 1994, p. 292). Music is often a universal language that many patients enjoy. Nurses can use music as a way of connecting heart to heart with patients.

VISUALIZATION AND IMAGERY

I once heard imagination defined as "I-magic" or "eye-magic." Imagination is the magic and power of vision, inner vision. Imagination is the fuel for the creative process. In my training as a dancer and choreographer, I was taught to use the power of my imagination, or inner sight, to recreate movement in my body as well as to create dances. Imagination or imagery is a creation of the mind. "Imagery is a flow of thoughts you can see, hear, feel, smell, or taste. An image is an inner representation of your experience or your fantasies—a way your mind codes, stores, and expresses information. Imagery is the currency of dreams and daydreams; memories and reminiscence; plans, projections, and possibilities. It is the language of the arts, the emotions and most important, of the deeper self" (Rossman, 1987, p. 14). The power of the mind expressed in the process of imagery can be used for healing.

Imagery allows us to have contact with our autonomic nervous system. Imagery can affect heart rate, respiratory patterns, gastrointestinal and brain wave patterns, and immune system function. Imagery is a *connection* between mind and body. In the search for understanding the power of imagery in healing, more has been learned about the function of the brain.

The Nobel Prize–winning work of Dr. Roger Sperry and other scientists has shown that the left and right brains have different functions in that they think in different ways. The left brain in most people thinks logically and is oriented around names and words. The left brain processes information sequentially. The right brain thinks in pictures, sounds, and feeling and processes information simultaneously. The right brain enables people to "see the whole picture" (Rossman, 1987, p. 19). Being able to see the bigger picture is what nurses often do with patients when providing support and education as to the "purpose" of the illness the patient is experiencing.

In Chapter 10, the patient experiencing a half-paralyzed esophagus was able to see the bigger picture and the purpose of her illness. The patient was able to use her right brain, her imagination, to "talk" her body's language and understand the meaning for her to have the condition. It was a very emotional moment for her when she realized the meaning of her illness—her conflicted feelings about placing her daughter in a foster home. "The right brain has a special relationship not only to imagery but to emotions. Many studies have shown that the right brain is specialized to recognize emotion in facial expressions, body language, speech, and even music. This is critical to healing because emotions are not only psychological but physical states that are at the root of a great deal of illness and disease" (Rossman, 1987, p. 21). Nurses who help patients deal with their disease through the use of imagery and visualization, help patients *connect* deeply with their body's memory, inner wisdom, and vital power.

MOVEMENT

Throughout my life I have seen the importance of movement as an indication of health, life, and spirit. When I talk about spirit, I mean the life force within all of us that is no respecter of gender, race, or religious belief. Spirit is the energy that beats our hearts and fills our lungs with air. How to be in touch with that spirit, or life force, was taught to me at a very young age in my dance classes. For the dancer, dance and movement are the externalization of spirit. It is the art of expressing the life force and the vital power Nightingale spoke of one hundred years ago.

Dance has been used by many cultures throughout history in religious and healing practices. African healers dance to bring forth the healing power within the sick. Dancers used healing movement patterns and gestures in the healing temples of India and Egypt. Today, dance therapists *connect* with some patients through movement when no other therapy is even remotely effective. I have used movement to communicate with the elderly and infants, as well as with autistic and developmentally challenged children.

Nurses continue to promote movement by turning patients and doing range-of-motion exercises. Nurses also promote movement on a cellular level by administering intravenous fluids and electrolytes. Whether large or small, all patient movement is important to the patient's health and healing. Some nurses are embracing the importance of movement and health and are expanding their practices to include movement modalities.

TAI CHI.   A colleague of mine studied tai chi in China. The senior center she manages has integrated tai chi into the program. Tai chi is a flowing, sustained, total-body exercise that is hundreds of years old and has been used by the Chinese to promote the flow of qi, or energy, throughout the body. Because it is believed in Eastern healing traditions that disease is caused by energy stagnation, it is also believed that by enhancing energy or chi movement throughout the body, health and longevity are promoted. Many of the seniors who study tai chi at my colleague's center toss aside their walkers after practicing tai chi.

YOGA.   Yoga is another movement modality. The word *yoga* is derived from the Sanskrit word meaning to "join." "The goal of the ancient tradition of yoga is the stilling of the restlessness of the mind and the joining of the mind, body, and spirit in the search for health, self-awareness, and spiritual attainment" (Collins, 1998, p. 564). To practice yoga postures and yoga breathing techniques that help calm and connect spirit, mind, and body, one does not have to subscribe to any particular religious belief or practice. One type of yoga breathing, for example, has been taught by labor and delivery nurses for years to women during childbirth.

TOUCH AND ENERGY FLOW.   In addition to movement itself as a modality, modalities that cause movement of energy are also used in nursing practice. Nurses use touch therapies such as massage, jin shin jyutsu and therapeutic touch to assist the smooth, rhythmic movement of energy throughout the patient's body. Often the patient experiences better sleep and an improved sense of well-being. Nurses who use these touch modalities to move energy spend years developing a sensitivity to the flow of energy in the body and to the multitude of differences in energy patterns that exist from patient to patient. Some nurses use touch therapies such as massage strictly for the physiological effect. Some nurses using these therapies are also aware of the energetic effects of the modality as well. Therapeutic touch in particular is one modality in which the practitioner's focus is more toward the energetic effect rather than the physiological touch effect. "The framework within which therapeutic touch continues to be researched, taught, and practiced postulates that people are open systems of energy and that an exchange of energy is the underlying dynamic by which TT has an effect" (Quinn, 1989, p. 79).

ELECTROTHERAPY.   Finally, electrotherapy, also found in historical nursing textbooks, was used to cause the movement of energy (i.e., stimulation or depression of tissue) and bring about chemical changes in cells, such as the rearrangement of ions, displacement of ions, or introduction of new ions from the outside (Parker, 1921). The field of electrotherapy was considered a specialization for physicians and nurses in the early 1900s just as radiology is today. Requirements for a registered nurse included, "Thorough, exact and accurate in her work, capable of careful and maintained attention and not easily excitable" (p. 322).

Some nurses today are involved in pain management in which they use transcutaneous electrical nerve stimulator (TENS) units. I used them on a surgical unit where we were able to decrease the amount of narcotic medication given to postoperative patients because of the use of TENS. I also had the opportunity to develop therapy protocols for electromagnetic devices used for low back pain and orthopedic injuries. Although at first quite skeptical, I found electromagnetic therapy, the use of electric current, to be highly effective for pain relief and the strengthening of muscles and joints.

Conclusion

All the modalities used in nursing deal with the patient's vital power or energy. Each of the modalities, from therapeutic touch, to TENS, to the administration of drugs, affects the patient's energy in different ways. More research and experience are needed in all areas. Energy is life; energy is vitality and vital power. It is human nature for patients to look for ways to live better and longer. These energy modalities have something to offer. Nurses must continue their historical practice of exploring the use of energy in the promotion of healing, health, and longevity. Resources for further learning about the use of energy in healing are provided in Appendix F.

References

Becker, R. (1990). *Cross currents.* Los Angeles, CA: Jeremy P. Tarcher, Inc.

Childre, D. L. (1994). *Freeze frame.* Boulder Creek, CA: Planetary Publications.

Chinn, P. L., & Watson, J. (1994). *Art and aesthetics in nursing.* New York: National League for Nursing.

Collins, C. (1998). Yoga: Intuition, preventive medicine, and treatment. *Journal of Obstetrics, Gynecology, & Neonatal Nursing, 27* (5), 563–568.

Davidson, A. W. (1988). *Choice patterns: A theory of the human-environment relationship.* Unpublished doctoral dissertation, University of Colorado, Denver.

Friedman, R., Sedler, M., Myers, P., & Benson, H. (1997). Behavioral medicine, complementary medicine, and integrated care: Economic implications. *Primary Care, 24* (4), 949–962.

Gerber, R. (1988). *Vibrational medicine.* Santa Fe, NM: Bear and Company.

Harmer, B. (1924). *Text-book of the principles and practice of nursing.* New York: Macmillan Co.

Knight, F., Wagner, C., & Chateris, M. (1889). *Medical facts concerning Colorado Springs.* Colorado Springs, CO: The Gazette Printing Company.

Merriam-Webster's collegiate dictionary. (10th ed.). (1993). Springfield, MA: Merriam-Webster.

Nightingale, F. (1957). *Notes on nursing.* Philadelphia: J.B. Lippincott Co.

Olson, S. (1998). Bedside musical care: Applications in pregnancy, childbirth, and neonatal care. *Journal of Obstetrics, Gynecology, & Neonatal Nursing, 27* (5), 569–575.

Parker, L. A. (1921). *Materia medica and therapeutics: A textbook for nurses.* Philadelphia: Lea and Febiger.

Quinn, J. F. (1989). Therapeutic touch as energy exchange: Replication and extension. *Nursing Science Quarterly, 2* (2), 79–87.

Rossman, M. (1987). *Healing yourself.* New York: Pocket Books.

Terman, M., Terman, J. S., & Ross, D. (1998). A controlled trial of timed bright light and negative air ionization for treatment of winter depression. *Archives of General Psychiatry, 55* (Oct), 875–882.

Tracy, M. (1938). *Nursing: An art and a science.* St. Louis, MO: C.V. Mosby Co.

Williams, S. (1993). Harp therapy: A psychoacoustic approach to treating pain and stress. *The American Harp Journal, 2,* 6–10.

Wirz-Justice, A. (1998). Beginning to see the light. *Archives of General Psychiatry, 55* (Oct), 861–862.

PART FOUR

THE EVOLUTION OF NURSING PRACTICE

NURSING PRACTICE HAS EVOLVED THROUGHOUT HISTORY. Whereas only fifty years ago, nurses might have had one type of touch therapy, such as massage, to learn and use in practice, today there are many modalities related to the health benefits of touch for them to learn and offer patients. Whereas years ago, being a nurse with good communication skills meant that the nurse was a good listener, today nurses take active roles in using various communication techniques to provide counseling to patients. Many historical nursing fundamentals are now "complementary therapies." These caring modalities are valuable offerings nurses bring to patient care.

Although simple, they can have a profound impact on the healing process and the healing relationship. The manner in which nurses care for patients is evolving. That evolution can take many forms and directions. The choices of those involved determine what direction the process of growth and change will take. Will nursing practice continue to model itself after the choices and practice of biomedicine? Will the lure of technology be so great that nurses completely disregard the opportunity to develop and research fundamental nursing care to pursue the values of the biomedical world and its "cures"? Will professional nurses continue to delegate or allow other professionals and unlicensed nursing assistants to perform those caring modalities that could be researched and developed by an educated professional nurse?

The modalities discussed in this book—the fundamentals of nursing practice used throughout history—can continue to provide a rich forum for research and development in professional nursing. There are numerous possibilities for developing the modalities of touch, use of environment, nutrition, communication, and energy in nursing practice. Clinical development, research, and creativity are needed to increase awareness and understanding of the importance of these fundamentals to patient care.

Integrative nursing is the creation of evolving, healing relationships with patients in which the nurse observes the patient's need for greater harmony and balance in life and then addresses that need by offering care that is a holistic blend of biomedical and caring modalities. It represents an opportunity for nurses to synthesize all that has developed as nursing practice over the years and put that knowledge to use in a new way, rather than having to choose between a practice in which only biomedical skills *or* caring skills are used. Integrative nursing represents a creative opportunity for all nurses to choose from the theories and holistic practices that make nursing unique and put together a plan of care that truly meets a patient's needs.

Evolution, development, and change are inevitable in nursing practice. Nursing is no different than any other service profession in that regard. People and societies evolve, develop, and change. Nurses must consider the ways to continue to meet society's demand and expectations for care. Many aspects of culture, including art, science, and healing, historically reflect the society's evolutionary process. The final chapters of this book discuss some key concepts involved in the evolutionary process.

Technologically developed nations are being challenged by their citizens to accept and integrate many paths of healing and health care. With the increase in world travel and the influence of the Internet, people in many nations are exposed to, and experimenting with, healing modalities and models of health care quite different from their own. *The public is practicing integrative care already!* People look for what works for their healing and health care needs. Contrary to popular scientific belief, most of the public is quite skeptical before trying something new. In my consultation practice, I receive many calls from people who want to make informed choices about their health care. Before calling me, they have been to their medical practitioners and have tried biomedical therapies alone. Many people continue to look for practitioners and therapies that will address all their needs related to a particular condition. Most people recognize that an ailment that makes them go to a doctor is often only a symptom. They want to be treated holistically, not just have the symptom go away.

I had a client whose seventeen-year-old son had begun having seizures when he turned sixteen. Because of the side effects, the mother did not like the idea of her son having to take seizure medication for the rest of his life. She asked me to consult with them about all their health care options, including the use of nonbiomedical therapies. This family needed a nurse to help them sort out all potential options for care and help them make the decision about the best course of action for the boy. The boy's physicians and alternative medicine practitioners were each presenting their views of what he should do. The family needed someone to help them integrate all the information and options and decide the best approach—an approach that would include learning and healing, not just removal of seizures. They knew that medication was a questionable "cure" and that they needed to find a path of healing and health care that used more than one approach; they wanted an integrative approach.

Nurses often perform the role of integrator of care. We help patients and their families identify their health needs and the choices they have of coping with a situation involving their health. From the choices that are made, a plan of *care* emerges. In the integrative model of nursing practice, the nurse uses keen observation and *heart* listening not only to identify patient and family needs so that she can formulate a plan of care with the patient, but also to develop a *relationship* with that patient. Relationship is the foundation for the nurse's involvement in patient care. Without some level of established relationship, the nurse can only speculate about the needs of the patient.

In an integrative model, the nurse's goal of relationship building is to come to an understanding of the ways in which the patient believes he can achieve greater balance (and a relationship) within his own being and with his environment. Balance also implies *relationship*. Balance is recognized in relation to something else. The nurse uses observation to gain greater understanding of the needs of the patient and then, as the healing relationship develops, interacts with the patient through the use of a holistic blend of various biomedical and caring modalities chosen by the patient to support the healing process. Nurses in healing relationships help patients not only to choose modalities of care but also to find *meaning* in the healing process itself.

Patients find meaning in many ways. The integrative nursing process provides an opportunity for the patient to find meaning in relationships—the relationship of the patient to himself and all that he is spiritually, emotionally, mentally, and physically; the relationship of the patient to the chosen healing or treatment modality; the relationship of the patient with his family, his community, his environment; and the relationship of the patient and the nurse who is also part of that environment. Relationship is connection. Healing occurs in relation and in connection, but rarely in isolation.

The quest for healing and health, and the desire for someone to help in the search, is a very human experience. People do not want to suffer alone; they look to health care providers to assist them with the changes they must go through to find better health. People who ask nurses for help are seeking a healing relationship that encompasses the concepts of holism, balance, compassion, and integration. An integrative nursing practice in which the core principle is relationship can provide the framework for patients engaging in a healing experience.

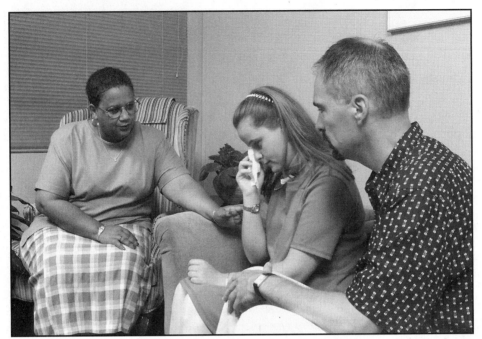

Nurse comforting couple in the 1990s

Compassion is the chief and perhaps only law of human existence.

—FYODOR DOSTOYEVSKY

CHAPTER 12

A Model for Integrative Nursing Practice

Nurses have performed the work of healing compassion side by side with practitioners who often have very different goals. Nurses have spent years developing working relationships with biomedical practitioners whose scientific concepts, values, and actions are very different. The relationship between nurses and physicians has changed in just a short period of time. The role of the nurse has evolved from that of handmaiden or servant to a partner to a colleague, especially with the emergence of nurses as primary care providers. I've had physician colleagues ask, "Do nurses want our jobs?" I've heard patients say, "The nurse is not a doctor. I want a doctor." Nurses are asking the same questions. "How am I different from my colleague, the physician? What do I offer the patient as a nurse?" Often nurses need to take time to step back from the world of biomedicine and reevaluate their practice and how it can develop as a separate yet parallel path to biomedicine. Nurses are at a crossroads of redefining what their relationship with other health care providers and patients is and can become.

Redefining relationships takes time and effort. There seem to be parallel processes occurring both between nurses and the biomedical world and between nurses and their patients. Whereas nurses are changing their role with biomedical practitioners to a level of partnership, patients are doing the same with nurses. Patients seek a partnership with their nurse. Nurses who take full responsibility and accountability for the healing of a patient, instead of developing partnerships with patients (or in the case of a child or comatose patient, a partnership with the family), can be "overcaring" and experience burnout. "Healing is personal and can only be facilitated by empowering the other person. The dictionary defines facilitate as 'to make easier, to assist the progress of a person.' This means a partnership; in other words, you are only part of the process" (Wells-Federman, 1996, p. 16). Nurses practicing from an integrative model facilitate and participate in a partnership with people seeking healing. Partnership is a relationship of compassion. Integrative nurses help patients find the best "condition," literally and figuratively, for nature to work; for the healing power within the *self* of the patient to come forth. Nature, the patient, loved ones, and the nurse engage in a healing partnership, a healing relationship.

Patients and their caregivers are given an opportunity to learn more about themselves by entering into a healing relationship. Drs. Hall and Allan wrote an article in 1994 called "Self in Relation" that eloquently portrays the joint quest for healing by patients and the nurses who care for them. They write, " Health is not something that one gives to someone else as much as it is a value shared between the client and the healer...the core of nursing practice is helping clients to fully use their sense of self as they cope with whatever changes they are finding in their physical, psychological, spiritual, and social worlds. This self is developed through relationship with practitioners whose holistic view of self and others allows the person to incorporate and expand this sense of self while engaging in decision making and holistic health practices. . . . The self is created in relation to others" (Hall & Allan, 1994, pp. 110, 112).

Finding and creating self is a way to find meaning in life. As a person learns more about himself, he develops an identity. When two people come together, both "selves" contribute to the building of the relationship. Nurses and patients both contribute to a healing relationship and therefore both can be *healed* by that relationship. That healing can manifest in many ways. It can be physical. It can mean gaining insight that rests a troubled mind. And it can mean having a spiritual experience. Healing is a life-changing event that is not easily forgotten. Healing is meaningful. Healing is a blessing to be had for all, including nurses. Healing, like communication, is a "two-way street" between nurse and patient. It can be a heart-to-heart, soul-to-soul experience in connection.

Connection

My first experience of a healing relationship and connection was not as a nurse but as a dancer. I was performing with Sachiyo Ito Dance Company in New York City. I had an experience that I will never be able to completely capture in words because it was an experience of the joy of connecting with the spirit of the dance and the energy flowing in my body as the instrument of the dance. As I performed this one dance, I felt a sense of peace, health, and wholeness. I was not separate from the dance anymore; I had become the dance. Through the experience, I somehow gained an understanding about myself and who I am deep inside—my identity—an inner knowledge I carry to this day. I had audience members say that they were profoundly moved, uplifted, and healed by the dance as well. Both the giver and the receiver of the dance were healed.

The same can happen in nursing. Both giver and receiver of healing can be healed in the process of connection. People are in a constant state of movement and adaptation. There is not a moment when we are not seeking balance at some level of our being. There is not a moment when we cannot benefit from the healing and balancing power of nature, love, or spirit. Nurses can benefit by being fully present, willing, and able to embrace the healing that emerges in each relationship with a patient. Patients and nurses are empowered by being in relationship with others. Each has potential to give and/or receive healing and to learn more about "self." "The relationship that is formed when clients and therapists are both empowered develops the self in both. The idea that the client must also be allowed the joy of helping the caring one discover himself or herself has been ignored because most of the theories that guide our care always depict an asymmetric and hierarchic arrangement between the nurse and the client, not an egalitarian and mutually empowering relationship" (Hall & Allan, 1994, pp. 113, 114).

The model, or visual diagram, used to depict the integrative nursing process is a geometric shape that exemplifies the importance of the balanced, mutually healing, and empowering relationship. This shape is present in every cell of our being. The shape of the double helix represented in human DNA is the model for integrative nursing (see Figure 12–1). Perhaps the double helix is represented in every cell of our being as a reminder from our creator that we, as human beings, and nurses are *about* relationship.

The Vision: Attaining the Double Helix

Using a nursing *model* in practice is similar to using a mission statement in an organization. The model and the mission statement are meant to provide a vision for those who work together for common goals. Models, like mission statements, don't get used unless they are meaningful and easy to articulate. For example, the starship crew on the American TV show "Star Trek" all know the mission of the starship Enterprise and are able to articulate it at any time, "To seek out new life and new civilizations . . . and to never violate the prime directive of noninterference with those civilizations."

Models and mission statements are meaningful in nursing if they provide support for decision making in practice. There are many highly thoughtful and relevant nursing models used in practice today. I have used many nursing models, including the Roy Adaptation Model for Nursing, which I studied for three years as part of my

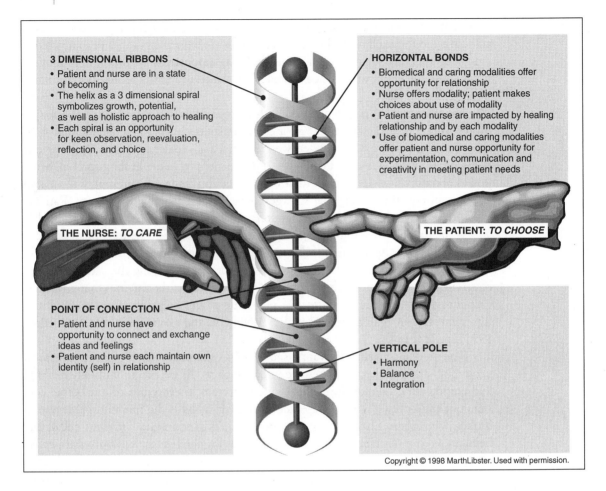

3 DIMENSIONAL RIBBONS
- Patient and nurse are in a state of becoming
- The helix as a 3 dimensional spiral symbolizes growth, potential, as well as holistic approach to healing
- Each spiral is an opportunity for keen observation, reevaluation, reflection, and choice

HORIZONTAL BONDS
- Biomedical and caring modalities offer opportunity for relationship
- Nurse offers modality; patient makes choices about use of modality
- Patient and nurse are impacted by healing relationship and by each modality
- Use of biomedical and caring modalities offer patient and nurse opportunity for experimentation, communication and creativity in meeting patient needs

THE NURSE: *TO CARE*

THE PATIENT: *TO CHOOSE*

POINT OF CONNECTION
- Patient and nurse have opportunity to connect and exchange ideas and feelings
- Patient and nurse each maintain own identity (self) in relationship

VERTICAL POLE
- Harmony
- Balance
- Integration

Copyright © 1998 MarthLibster. Used with permission.

FIGURE 12–1
Healing relationship model for integrative nursing

nursing education. The visual model for integrative nursing in Figure 12–1 is a symbolic representation of the development of the healing *relationship* as a core value and possible mission "statement" for nursing practice. The two ribbons and horizontal bars of the double helix itself serve as a metaphor for the nurse-patient relationship representing two, multidimensional beings in relationship. The double helix model can be used as a focal point and a reminder that the goal of the nursing process is to create evolving, healing relationships. Having this as a vision and mission is important when nurses make important decisions about patient care, when they decide what the focus of nursing education should be, and when they decide what direction nursing practice will take.

Caring, like healing, does not occur in isolation. Caring occurs between two or more people. The image of the nurse engaging in caring acts serves as an example to society of the importance of human contact and demonstrating care to self and others. Nurses also serve as reminders of the relationship to a higher healing power as they put the patient in the best condition for nature to work upon him. The double helix and the healing relationship model is symbolic of a nursing practice where compassionate, healing relationships are formed that enable adaptation and greater balance of spirit, mind, and body to occur.

NURSES IN RELATION

The geometric design known as the double helix is represented throughout the human body in every cell. It is represented in the structure known as deoxyribose nucleic acid or DNA. DNA is composed of two helical-shaped chains each coiled around the same axis. In the integrative nursing model (Figure 12–1) the helixes represent the nurse and the patient. Both have the same "axis," and focus—healing.

The helix is a clear expression of the healing process. The helix, like the healing process, is not a straight line, circle, or spiral. Healing is not linear. People remember their health concerns, they do not just move on, as a straight line, without ever revisiting the concern. For example, the person who is burned in fire has a constant reminder in the scar tissue. People who take medication for chronic pain remember and reenact, on a daily basis, the beneficial effects of their pain medication so that they can function their best in society. Healing is not circular. Although some people may feel as if they are sometimes going around in circles during the healing process, they do indeed grow all the time, even in small ways, in the knowledge of their illness or health concern as well as in their ability to face their health concern. Healing isn't really a spiral-shaped process either. People do reevaluate, or "spiral" back to revisit and rethink the decisions made during the healing and learning process. For example, a surgical patient walks for the first time and goes a short distance. She feels good, so the next day she increases the distance. But sometimes she goes too far and experiences an increase in pain and shortness of breath. This is like a spiral; she circles back after reflecting on the healing process and realizes that she did too much. The next day she doesn't walk as far. This experience in the healing process is not like the two-dimensional spiral. The patient grows throughout the experience. The multi-dimensional, vertically expanded helix is a better visual expression of how the patient and caregivers grow or evolve in understanding the healing process unique to the individuals in the healing relationship.

The healing process is at least three-dimensional, with multiple turns like the helix. At each "curve" in the process, assessments, interventions, and/or evaluations are made by the nurse and patient and something is learned, such as whether or not the modality used in nursing care was helpful to the individual. As learning takes place, both the patient and the nurse learn more about themselves and each other,

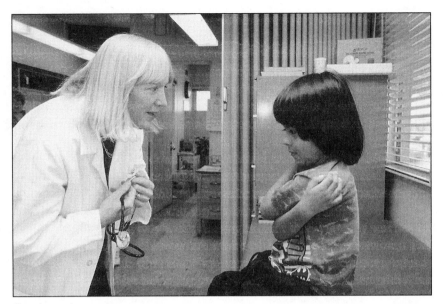

Creating an impression

and what each brings to the healing relationship. They grow and move forward. The helix represents the integration process in that it demonstrates the cycling back on itself, but never goes back to the exact point of origin. Both helices maintain their multidimensional movement on their own course in relation to the other helix. The double helix as a model for integrative nursing demonstrates the healing relationship of two, multidimensional beings who are in a constant state of balance, growth, and learning.

Human DNA is composed of different strings of molecules called nucleotides. Depending upon their chemical composition, these nucleotides are connected in a ladderlike pattern of horizontal bonds to other nucleotides within the structure of the DNA. Each helix "relates" to the other in the double helix design. The relationship of one helix to another is represented by the horizontal bonds. In the healing relationship model for integrative nursing practice, the horizontal bonds symbolize the human connection, compassion, contact, and caring shared between the patient and the nurse.

ENCODING, MEMORY, AND IMPRESSIONS

Nurses, through their work with patients, not only create healing relationships, they also create memory. Both the nurse and the patient become part of the memory of each other. The healing relationship, as with all life experiences and interactions with environment, is *encoded* upon our cells, our DNA. Encoding is the first stage of the memory process where information is taken in. "This is followed by storage and retrieval, involving processes associated with receiving or briefly registering stimuli through one or more senses and modifying that information" (Stedman's Medical Dictionary, 1990). Whether or not an experience is stored in memory, be it long or short term, is a very complex process. The emotional nature of the event has a lot to do with how the event is remembered. "Emotion may either enhance memory (hypermnesia) or impair memory (hypomnesia) and occasionally even create a 'curious combination of both these effects'" (Cahill, 1999, p. 239). Extreme stress or trauma significantly affects the experience of a patient and the healing experience. If the nurse-patient experience is perceived as traumatic rather than healing, balancing, and energizing, the body might store the memory of the relationship as "traumatic." The patient would then experience a stress response, which, as discussed in previous chapters, decreases the ability of the body to attend to healing and balance. The stress response takes energy away from the healing process.

Not only do nurses create healing, stress-free environments with patients, but also they have the opportunity to create powerful memories of a positive healing experience with the patients and for themselves as well. Traumatic memories are draining for everyone. Difficult health care situations do not have to be traumatic. Nurses are often the only ones who work to prevent a patient's potential trauma reaction. For example, hospitalization can be extremely traumatic for anyone. No one wants to be sick, at a low point energetically in his life, and be in a strange, uncomfortable environment. This can quickly register as "trauma." Nurses help the patient adapt to the hospital environment to promote healing. Many patients encode and remember the kindness and attention of the nurse long after the hospital experience is over.

Life experiences such as hospitalization and an interaction with a nurse are recorded, so to speak, in the being of the patient. The patient learns about the healing relationship through his experiences with healing people and environments. The learning process includes the sensory experience of the interface of the patient's nervous system with the environment. "Inherited neuronal connections determine the range of things it will be possible to learn, and changes in the basic activity of key neurons in response to life experience can shift the balance between intricate networks of neurons to make certain mental and physical events more or less prominent. . . . Our genetic equipment therefore is modified by experience throughout the life span" (Dubovsky, 1997, p. 69).

Creating a healing environment and being caring toward patients is not just good nursing practice, nor is it just good customer service. The healing relationship of the nurse and the patient is *remembered.* The relationship may even indirectly modify the genetic makeup of the persons involved for good or for ill. The healing relationship has incredible power and influence on the health and well-being of people and, potentially, a civilization. Nurses must recognize the importance of their commitment to understanding and enhancing the healing relationship and all the caring modalities that influence it. Nurses have the opportunity to help patients create powerful memories of peaceful, healing experiences. It takes effort, care, and love, but more than this, it takes the realization by nurses themselves that what they do and who they are when they provide care to patients is powerful and is vitally important to health, life, and perhaps even human evolution and survival.

CARING CAN BE LEARNED

Caring is learned by experience. Nurses care for patients who then have the opportunity to remember, or learn, what it means to be cared for. Learning involves memory and processing experience. Nurses also learn through experience what it means to be and feel caring and how to demonstrate caring. Caring *can* be learned and taught.

Caring is a virtue, a way of being, as well as an action or behavior. "Most moral philosophers do not regard virtues as inborn personality traits or dispositions over which people have no control and for which they have minimal responsibility" (Brody, 1988, p. 89). People learn caring and compassion by receiving and experiencing caring and compassion. The goal of learning or teaching caring must be *experiencing* care. Nurses who want to learn to care as a professional goal need to have a variety of experiences in giving and receiving care.

There are as many ways of caring as there are healing relationships. Healing relationships determine the nature of the care that is received and given. Each nurse must find her own approach to caring. "Knowledge cannot be given to another. We can expose our students to a body of information but only they, by their own intellectual work of figuring out and coming to terms with the logic of that information, can transform it into knowledge. . . . Each nurse gains knowledge about nursing practice in such a way that every clinical experience becomes a lesson which informs the next practice experience" (Paul & Heaslip, 1995, pp. 40–41). Nurses learn caring by experiencing what it is like to be a part of a caring, healing relationship. Each patient's relationship with a nurse is unique. Each unique relationship gives the nurse another chance to learn what it means to be and act caring. Learning what it means to be caring is an ongoing, cumulative process, that can continue for a lifetime.

Because caring is an expression and experience of relationship, it is difficult to identify precisely what a caring behavior is. For example, Forsyth, Delaney, Maloney, Kubesh, and Story define caring as the "nonverbal components of therapeutic interaction" (1989). They discuss both the nonverbal "component" and its associated "characteristics" of caring. The first component listed is "openness" and the related characteristics listed are "open body posture, eye contact and alertness to patient needs" (p. 166). Alertness to patient needs is a general concept of integrative nursing that can be applied to any healing relationship; however, the first two characteristics are highly situational. For example, some cultures find it highly offensive to have eye contact with someone. While caring for a nine-year-old boy with severe behavioral problems related to his developmental delays I learned very quickly that an open body posture and eye contact were, at certain times (such as when setting a limit) not caring. I had to cross my arms and look away from him so that he would understand that his behavior was inappropriate. If I looked at him in an open posture he would laugh. This child taught me that there are no absolutes when it comes to determining what caring behavior is. Caring is defined by the individuals experiencing the relationship.

In learning to care, nurses build a "memory bank" of caring experiences to draw from when creating relationships with patients. The double helix reminds us that, like DNA with its genetic coding, we are creating memories. Nurses need learning experiences that open their hearts and minds to the sensations of caring experience.

Nurses who have never experienced being cared for can have difficulty comprehending what it means to care for someone else. Nurse educators have the opportunity and responsibility to expose student nurses to the many aspects of caring behavior and caring modalities, the role of caregiver, and care receiver. The process of developing the virtue of being a caring human being involves learning to be both a caregiver and a care receiver.

The movie *The Doctor* exemplified this way of teaching and learning caring. The physician in the movie is detached from his patients and his family until he is diagnosed with cancer. The movie depicts his health care experience as cold and impersonal. The doctor finds ways of getting his caring needs met outside of the biomedical world. He survives his cancer experience to become an educator of medical students. During clinical rotations he exposes his students to every test they would ever prescribe for a patient. The students quickly come up with ways to demonstrate caring for others during the treatment because they experience firsthand what is uncomfortable about the procedure. The students in the movie experienced an enema or having blood drawn. People who have gone through a healing crisis themselves and have been on the receiving end of care often make very caring, compassionate health care providers. Caring is learned through many professional and life experiences.

As a nursing student I had the opportunity to work in a foot reflexology clinic for two years. I learned about caring through the use of touch in a way that I did not in the classroom. I learned that touch could be used therapeutically, not just procedurally. I learned about caring in a way that was different from what I learned in my skills lab in nursing school. I have taught foot reflexology for many years and have found that the people who attend the class have a deeply moving experience of what it is like to be cared for and what it is like to care for someone else by caring for their feet. Learning caring modalities such as touch therapies provides nurses the opportunity to develop the art and skill of demonstrating care.

Through the ongoing nursing process of assessment, interaction/intervention, and evaluation, a nurse receives constant feedback on whether what she is doing is perceived as caring. Nurses are responsible for their ability to meet the caring needs of patients. Even nurses who develop extensive repertoires of biomedical skills and caring modalities, such as complementary therapies, are not necessarily going to be perceived by patients as caring. Techniques, skills, instruments, and modalities are only a means to an end. That end is the healing relationship that provides the nurse with a foundation from which she can better identify effective ways of meeting the caring needs of patients. Providing care is an ongoing learning process that occurs in relationships with patients.

"Measuring" the Outcome

It has become common for nurses to be asked to validate, and sometimes justify, the caring work they perform with patients. There are many reasons for this, often related to allocation of resources. Money is given to programs that are valued by those in control of the resources. For example, new mothers used to remain in the hospital for a few days of rest and recuperation after giving birth. Apart from the fact that many women prefer to recuperate at home, many insurance companies in the West no longer recognize any value to a mother being hospitalized beyond two days postpartum. Some value is placed on mothers receiving a nurse visit in the home, but not all insurance companies allow for this service. There are many health care issues such as this that demand that nurses justify their caring role in the health care of patients.

Measuring the impact and importance of nursing care to the patient's health and well-being is not an easy matter. Alternate research methods to the standard quantitative methods of exploration may be helpful. But when all is said and done, the ultimate outcome or effectivity of nursing care is really "measured," or better yet evaluated, by the patient and the nurse themselves. The professional nurse may also find that the care they provide is highly individualized and difficult to measure in comparison to the healing experiences with other patients. Nurses must learn ways to "measure" the effectiveness of nursing care relative to the uniqueness of the individual patient.

SPIRALS OF CHANGE

Healing relationships are evolving, upward-spiraling *processes* in which nurses and patients do not know the outcome. The patient does know that he enters the relationship seeking assistance, care, support, education, and advice about health care decisions he must make and carry out. For example, a patient who experiences a major whiplash in a motor vehicle accident can try for years to cure his back and neck pain using multiple biomedical modalities. He can have back surgery and take strong pain and muscle spasm relieving medication for years. Relief can be minimal and he may not be able to hold a job. His family members may get frustrated with his daily complaints and inability to interact with them. The patient may get to a point where he is no longer helped by medicine. Nurses who pattern their practice after the medical model may not be able to help this man either. Nurses and health practitioners in pain clinics are often able to help patients such as this man learn to live with pain as opposed to focusing on extinguishing the pain. They do this by using techniques such as meditation and relaxation. Nursing work does not end with the relief of pain or the quieting of a distressful symptom. Patients such as the man with the whiplash pain always seek greater comfort, wellness, and wholeness. Where a practitioner of medicine might pronounce a patient as "healed" and the health care relationship ended when the symptom ends, the nursing process and the nurse-patient relationship often continue. This is especially evident in the practice of community and outpatient care.

As with the motion of the double helix, the nurse and patient experience many turns and spirals in their ongoing relationship. These spirals represent opportunities for assessment, evaluation, and reevaluation of care and wellness level. In the case of the man with the chronic back pain, the nurse and patient evaluate the patient's response to medical treatment, which may be effective initially at alleviating the pain. If the pain or health concern continues to be an issue, the nurse and patient then reevaluate the choices the patient has made for dealing with his pain. The nurse may guide the patient to explore what other modalities might be helpful. The nurse enters the world of the patient as she begins to create the healing relationship with the goal of meeting the patient where she is, not where she "should" be. The nurse provides options and resources as well as interventions. The nurse maintains an open mind to exploring all possible modalities and interventions to help the patient achieve greater balance, harmony, and wellness.

The patient and the healing relationships he has with a nurse are living *systems,* which by remaining "open" rather than "closed," allow for an exchange of information. Positive change and adaptation can occur when the dynamic process of the exchange of energy and information is present within the lives of the individuals involved in relationship. This positive change does not have to manifest as a "cure." Healing does not always include a cure or the eradication of illness. Because the nurse-patient relationship is an open system, the nurse stays in relationship with the patient throughout the healing process whether or not the patient experiences a cure. One nurse theorist, Dr. Betty Neuman, defines a system as "a pervasive order that holds together its parts" (1995, p. 8). She goes on to describe nursing as being a system "conceptualized as a complete whole with identifiable smaller wholes or parts. The whole structure is maintained by inter-relationships of system components, through regulations that evolve out of the dynamics of the open system. . . . Wholism is both a philosophical and biological concept, implying relationships and processes arising from wholeness, dynamic freedom, and creativity in adjusting to stressors in the internal and external environment" (p. 10).

Neuman's system theory provides a framework for conceptualizing the dynamic relationships within systems such as the relationship between the patient and the environment, with the nurse as a recognized part of that environment. As is expressed by the double helix, the patient and nurse continue to grow and evolve. That process of growth is affected by environment.

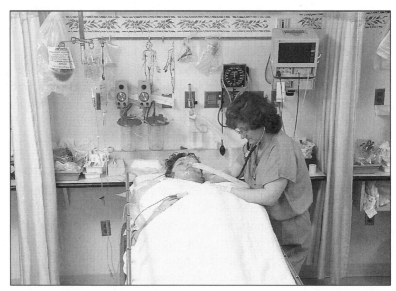

Demonstrating care in the PACU

Systems theory also describes the growth of a system. The patient as a system can experience entropy, "energy moving toward extinction . . . gradual disorganization and energy dissipation, or he can experience negentropy, absorbing energy to increase organization as he develops toward a steady or wellness state" (Neuman, 1995, p. 11). Both the healing relationship model, with its spiraling action, and systems theory depict nursing care as a flow of energy within the environment of the healing relationship. Neuman says that both the nurse, as part of the environment, and the patient are in an "exchange" process. "Nursing is primarily concerned with defining appropriate action in stress-related situations or in possible reactions of the client/client system; since environmental exchanges are reciprocal, both client and environment may be positively or negatively affected by each other" (p. 11). Nurses and their patients are part of a dynamic system with the healing relationship at the center. Like any system, healing relationships are not necessarily better understood by teasing out the individual parts that make up the whole. It is often more enlightening to study the whole. As nurses seek greater understanding about the process of caring, it is important to remember that the sum of the parts of any relationship is not necessarily greater than the relationship as a whole. In trying to evaluate the effects of nursing practice on people's lives, nurses are continually faced with the possibility that the outcome of their relationships with patients may not be measurable from a two- or even a three-dimensional perspective. Is it even possible to adequately "measure" the outcome of the dynamic, ongoing, energetic process of relationship?

EVIDENCE-BASED PRACTICE: THE BURDEN OF PROOF

If we knew what it was we were doing,
it would not be called research, would it?

—ALBERT EINSTEIN

Recently, there has been an increase in the emphasis in medicine and nursing to focus efforts on developing research utilization models for practice, known as evidence-based practice. The goal is to encourage the use of "evidence" in clinical decision making. Physicians, and now nurses, are promoting the use of "evidence." Evidence is defined as proof (Merriam-Webster's Collegiate Dictionary, 1999). The concept in science of finding evidence or proof is not new. Columbus wanted proof that the world was flat so he began mapping, calculating distance, and ultimately courageously sailing to what should have been the end of the earth. Of course, he found a new world in the process.

"Proof" is shaped by environment. Science seeks proof that is unbiased and unaffected by the seeker; science seeks objectivity. Hence the creation of the double blind, placebo controlled, clinical trial. But not all scientific questions can be answered with the double blind, placebo controlled trial, especially when human beings are involved. What is evidence, anyway, and who determines what is evidence?

Medicine took the lead on the introduction of evidence-based medicine (EBM). "An initial goal of EBM, it appears, was to minimize the use of non-evidentiary knowledge and reasoning in clinical practice" (Tonelli, 1998, p. 1235). Medicine has defined evidence-based medicine as using the knowledge gained from research in practice. Medical practitioners have already realized that to exclusively emphasize EBM as the "right" way to practice medicine is ineffective. Physicians do not accept being told that they *must* use the results/evidence of a particular study in the care of their patient.

Western physicians continue to resist the "cookbook" approach to medicine spawned by a managed care system. "EBM and managed care share a common epistemological focus on outcomes measured across populations" (Tonelli, 1998, p. 1238). Physicians value research, but they also value the patient's experience as well as their own clinical expertise. They use many forms of knowledge in clinical situations. The definition of EBM has been evolving. "More recently the focus [of EBM] has shifted to *integrating* clinical expertise, pathophysiologic knowledge, and patient preferences in making decisions regarding the care of individual patients. . . . The difficulty, then, becomes defining the appropriate situations when other forms of knowledge and reasoning take precedence" (p. 1235).

Nurses may want to learn from the experience of medicine regarding the evolution of evidence-based practice. "Evidence-based nursing de-emphasizes ritual, isolated and unsystematic clinical experiences, ungrounded opinions and tradition as a basis for nursing practices...and stresses instead the use of research findings and, as appropriate, quality improvement data, other operational and evaluation data, the consensus of recognized experts and affirmed experience to substantiate practice" (Stetler et al., 1998, p. 48). Nurses, like physicians, must reserve the right to practice their profession and make clinical judgments with patients based on many ways of knowing, including patient preference and the nurse's experience and expertise. Some nurse leaders have said, "How do we get nurses to use research?" rather than "How do we provide nurses with research so that they can choose whether or not to use it with a particular patient?" Hinshaw writes that research should be "transferred and used in the sense of principles and concepts and not in terms of procedures and standardized rules" (1989, p. 170). Evidence-based practice should not be allowed to become a mandate to professional nurses as the gold standard of clinical decision making.

Evidence-based nursing, like evidence-based medicine, is one type of knowledge that nurses bring to their work with patients. Sometimes the implication exists among some nurses that all nursing "should" be evidence based. As with other evolutions in nursing practice, there seem to be some who would throw the "baby out with the bath water" just because there are new ways to research and understand nursing practice. What happens to the expertise of the individual professional nurse?

Nursing research can be helpful to patient care. Yet, without the connection to the nurse-patient relationship, the use of research can become rote and the care of the individual human being mechanized. It is worrisome that some nurses would consider linking nursing research to the policies and procedures of health care institutions, thereby forcing nurses, who agree to follow the policies and procedures of the institution, to use the "evidence" whether or not it is appropriate for the patient. It is easy to see why most nurses might agree that a policy and procedure based on research on the use of saline rather than heparin for the maintenance of a capped IV line would be helpful. But if the standard were to link *all* nursing policies and procedures, including the use of caring modalities, to "evidence," nurses may be effectively stopped from providing care at all.

"Evidence based medicine is not 'cook-book' medicine. Because it requires a bottom-up approach that integrates the best external evidence with individual clinical expertise and patient choice, it cannot result in slavish, cook-book approaches to individual patient care. External clinical evidence can inform, but can never replace, individual clinical expertise and it is this expertise that decides whether the external evidence applies to the individual patient at all and, if so, how it should be integrated into the clinical decision" (Sackett, Richardson, Rosenberg, & Haynes, 1998, p. 3). Policy and procedure manuals are like cookbooks. With the tremendous growth in patient services and nursing activities, many institutions no longer write "cookbook" policies for nursing care. In addition to nurses using their own reference texts and journals to develop guidelines for practice, most institutions provide committee approved resources that nurses can use for reference within that institution. Nurses can use research as it emerges, and when it seems appropriate, and still maintain their right as a professional to make clinical decisions with patients with whom they have engaged in a healing relationship.

The healing relationship allows the nurse and patient to access different ways of knowing that support clinical decision making. John Wolfer, Ph.D., writes about the importance of different ways of knowing in nursing. He says, "All of these modes of knowing will be needed to improve the quality of caring for the whole patient (and the whole nurse). In other words, this map offers a way of looking at the reality of nursing which 'sees' different types of knowledge theory and research as complementary rather than competitive or exclusionary" (1993, p. 145). Although he is specifically discussing the different research methodologies available to researchers, this statement rings true for all types of knowledge in nursing. A complete appreciation, respect, and honoring of all types of knowing is needed. Heavy reliance on evidence or proof, and subtle condemnation of any nurse/patient clinical decision not based on "the evidence" from those not involved directly in the healing relationship, is a threat to the very foundation and values of professional nursing.

Nurses do not make decisions *for* patients. Nurses make decisions *with* patients. Our profession has a reputation for making shared decisions. This is because we value the healing relationship. Part of our way of "knowing" is to ask patients what they "know" and want. Disregard of patients' experiences can become part of our measurement-oriented health care system. "Administrators seek to control nursing actions, to limit caring time, and to require concrete, measurable outcomes, while nurses beg for time for caring tasks (listening to patient concerns) that do not have solid, quantifiable outcomes other than patient satisfaction" (Morse, 1989, as qtd. in Koch, 1994, p. 1150). When patients are asked to express their concerns in open-style interviews, one most striking feature is the emphasis on the importance of being acknowledged as an individual" (Koch, 1994, p. 1150). As nurses explore the expansion of evidence-based nursing practice, we must realize that because of our professional values, and the fact that most of the members of our profession practice in huge group practices (i.e., hospitals), it is a considerable challenge to promote the integration of the use of "evidence" with knowledge that emerges from the healing relationship in patient care. Integration of the concept of evidence-based practice into nurses' work has its limitations. Ethical dilemmas can occur as well.

Medicine has recognized the potential unfavorable consequences of misunderstanding evidence-based practice and failing to understand its limitations. The "untoward" consequences envisioned could also apply in nursing practice. Tonelli identifies limitations of evidence-based practice as, "The devaluation of the individual, a shift in the focus of practice from the individual to society at large, and the failure to appreciate and cultivate the complex nature of sound clinical judgement" (1998, p. 1237).

Lest any reader think that I am "against" EBM, let me say clearly, that I am *for* integration. The focus of integration is to encourage nurses to use all ways of knowing that might have relevance to a patient's care. Nurses can change the way they make clinical decisions by *adding* evidence to practice. Just as in medicine, the freedom of choice to use information gleaned from research must stay with the nurse and the patient. Nurses can benefit from more freedom and autonomy in practice, not less. Nurses need support in integrating all ways of knowing into practice. They should never be forced to choose one form of knowing over another by nurses in positions of power acting as "thought police." This is unscientific and biased. I would agree with Dr. Clark Smith, who in an editorial wrote, "I would not disagree that we need to pursue rational justification for the things we do in medicine. I think we must also guard against the elitist (and usually academic) view that if practice or a method or treatment can't be proved with a scientifically designed study and if we can't get the important data into our computers to manipulate, then somehow that method or practice is less worthy because that attitude itself is unscientific and cultist" (1997, p. 77). Smith writes in support of the *art* of medicine. Nursing is also an art. EBM must be integrated with the art of nursing, not placed in opposition to it. Art does not need proof or evidence. Much of what makes art enjoyable is its beauty and the often seeming purposelessness of it. Art comes from the heart and often finds no justification, let alone evidence; however, just as in science, art can be learned.

In the East, art is taught by master artists. The master artists teach by example rather than by lecture. Eugen Herrigel writes of his experience in Japan of learning the art of archery in his book, *Zen in the Art of Archery.* He learns from his master teacher that, "The right art is purposeless, aimless! The more obstinately you try to learn how to shoot the arrow for the sake of hitting the goal, the less you will succeed in the one and the further the other one will recede. What stands in your way is that you have a much too willful will. You think that what you do not do yourself does not happen" (Herrigel, 1971, p. 34). This sounds so much like Florence Nightingale and her instruction to "put the patient in the best condition possible for nature to work upon him." Healing is not only in our hands . . . we have the grace of being the witnesses to the healing experiences of others. We sometimes have the honor of being the instrument of healing. No one can "measure" the spirit of nursing, the healing spirit that arises in the relationship between nurse and patient. As nurses pursue greater use of research and evidence in practice, let us make sure that there will be an equally important place in nursing practice and education for the art and spirit of healing and the knowledge that comes out of the nurse-patient relationship.

Conclusion

We can find ways of integrating all ways of knowing when making decisions with patients. A clinical decision in nursing emerges as a result of the growing relationship between the patient and nurse. Decisions can be made in regard to the science/evidence, the spirit/art, as well as any influential administrative constraints. The science/evidence includes the nursing assessment, relevant research, and the knowledge and understanding of the patient and the nurse. The spirit/art includes the personal and clinical experiences of both the patient and the nurse, their personal values, cultural beliefs, and education. Administrative constraints include time, finances, community standards, policies, and laws. The nurse is very careful not to impose upon or make a decision *for* a patient. She gathers the information, options, and possibilities for care and shares in the decision making process with the patient. Regarding EBM, nurses know that, no amount of empiric health care data can ever dictate what a nurse or patient *ought* to do in any particular situation. Many nurses learn to develop the art and skill of shared decision making and help patients make health decisions they will remember without regret.

Chapter 13 discusses how nurses make clinical decisions with patients, how experience affects clinical decision making in nursing practice, and the process of how nurses choose from a repertoire of caring modalities.

References

Brody, J. (1988). Virtue ethics, caring, and nursing. *Scholarly Inquiry for Nursing Practice: An International Journal, 2* (2), 87–96.

Cahill, L. (1997). The neurobiology of emotionally influenced memory. *Annals of the New York Academy of Sciences, 821,* 238–246.

Dubovsky, S. (1997). *Mind body deceptions.* New York: W.W. Norton & Co.

Forsyth, D., Delaney, C., Maloney, N., Kubesh, D., & Story, D. (1989). Can caring behavior be taught? *Nursing Outlook, 37* (4), 164–166.

Hall, B. A., & Allan, J. D. (1994). Self in relation: A prolegomenon for holistic nursing. *Nursing Outlook, 15* (3), 110–116.

Herrigel, E. (1971). *Zen in the art of archery.* New York: Vintage Books.

Hinshaw, A. S. (1989). Nursing science: The challenge to develop knowledge. *Nursing Science Quarterly, 2* (4), 162–171.

Koch, T. (1994). Beyond measurement: Fourth-generation evaluation in nursing. *Journal of Advanced Nursing, 20,* 1148–1155.

Merriam-Webster's collegiate dictionary (10th ed.). (1999). Springfield, MA: Merriam-Webster.

Morse, J. (1989). *Qualitative nursing research: A contemporary dialogue.* Rockville, MD: Aspen.

Neuman, B. (1995). *The Neuman systems model* (3rd ed.). Norwalk, CT: Appleton & Lange.

Paul, R., & Heaslip, P. (1995). Critical thinking and intuitive nursing practice. *Journal of Advanced Nursing Practice, 22,* 40–47.

Sackett, D. L., Richardson, W. S., Rosenberg, W., & Haynes, R. B. (1998). *Evidence-based medicine: How to practice and teach EBM.* Edinburgh: Churchill Livingstone.

Smith, C. (1997). Evidence-based medicine and the art of medicine. *Journal of American Board of Family Practice, 10* (1), 76–77.

Stedman, T. (1990). *Stedman's medical dictionary* (25th ed.). Baltimore, MD: Williams & Wilkins.

Stetler, C. B., Brunell, M., Giuliano, K., Morsi, D., Prince, L., & Newell-Stokes, V. (1998). Evidence-based practice and the role of nursing leadership. *Journal of Nursing Administration, 28* (7/8), 45–53.

Tonelli, M. (1998). The philosophical limits of evidence-based medicine. *Academic Medicine, 73* (12), 1234–1240.

Wells-Federman, C. (1996). Awakening the nurse healer within. *Holistic Nursing Practice, 10* (2), 13–29.

Wolfer, J. (1993). Aspects of "reality" and ways of knowing in nursing: In search of an integrating paradigm. *Image, 25* (2), 141–146.

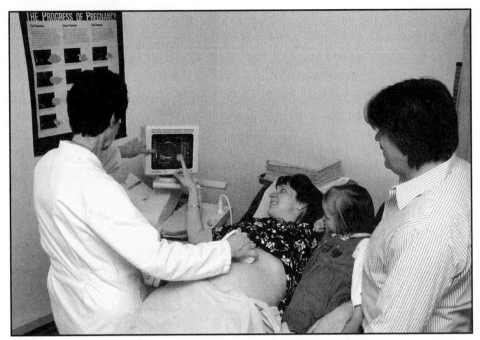

A nurse sharing a family experience

*Happiness is a perfume which you cannot pour on someone
without getting some on yourself.*

—Ralph Waldo Emerson

Choosing Caring Modalities

Chapters 1–12 discuss the importance of caring modalities, the importance of nurses continuing the historical tradition of expanding the science and art of caring in everyday practice with patients, and holding the vision of our method of practice as being founded in the development of the healing relationship. Not unlike the DNA in every cell of our being, we can demonstrate in our healing relationships the ability to harmonize, entrain, and perhaps even bond with another person while maintaining our own "helical" path. Having spoken of the underlying value of nursing as the healing relationship, a relationship that is unique with each and every patient, we turn now to the *actions* in the expression of that relationship. We've discussed how nurses demonstrate caring and what modalities she uses. Now we turn to *how* the nurse makes the decision to use a particular caring modality. How does the nurse *know* what modality to offer a patient?

Choosing a biomedical modality is often quite simple, although the actual process of implementation takes incredible skill. For example, a dehydrated patient needs to be rehydrated. The nurse has two choices—oral hydration or intravenous hydration. Depending on her assessment of the patient and her collaboration with the physician, the nurse will choose to force fluids and/or start an IV. If she decides to start an IV she must then address the next decision, which is often more complex. She must answer the question, "How will this patient respond to having an IV started and receiving lots of fluids?" A seemingly simple question, but let's just imagine for a moment that the patient is a five-day-old infant. The trauma of starting an IV in an infant who is dehydrated is significant for the baby, the family, and the nurse. *How* the nurse decides to care for the baby *and* the anxious parents involves choices about the use of caring modalities. Some of the questions the nurse might address are: How will she explain the procedure (communication techniques) to the infant's parents to be sure that the parents agree with the procedure and are willing to give informed consent? Will she use a warm water pack to the infant's extremity to help bring out the vein (hydrotherapy/environmental care)? Will she use therapeutic touch at the IV site after starting the IV to minimize pain from the insertion (touch therapy/use of energy)? The list of options goes on. The choices of caring modalities used are what constitute the art and science of caring. The choices are based on many ways of knowing, including research data, the nurse's clinical experience and expertise, and the patient's experiences and desires.

The example of starting an IV on an infant is an opportunity to practice *integrative nursing.* I have experimented in my own practice with just starting an IV without observing the patient or family needs or considering the blending of caring modalities. I have found that my rapport with patients and their families, as well as my experience of the nursing intervention, was very different depending on my approach. Observant integrative nurses realize that veins in a dehydrated infant are fragile and that increasing blood flow to the IV site through the use of warm, moist heat or therapeutic touch might help ease the insertion of the IV. Integrative nurses realize that an IV poke can cause stress that, in turn, can have an impact on the overall healing process even at a cellular level. Integrative nurses who are keenly observant know that the infant feels pain or discomfort from the procedure and might be comforted by being held by the parents as soon as possible after the procedure.

Am I discussing the obvious? I don't think so. There are some nurses who do not value providing caring modalities with every IV, every biomedical skill, and every nursing action. Caring modalities and the choice to use them takes skill, knowledge, expertise, and heart. Many nurses develop their own caring modalities over years of practice. There are many silent experts in nursing.

Expertise and Decision Making

Being able to integrate nursing knowledge and caring modalities requires a certain level of experience and expertise. To use the analogy of the cook once again . . . the cook cannot adjust a recipe until they learn the fundamentals of cooking. For example, a cook realizes the influence of humidity on the ability of bread to rise. A novice cook might follow a bread recipe to the letter, put the ingredients for the bread together, and start to knead the dough never realizing that the dough is not the right consistency due to excessive atmospheric humidity. This is because they have never made bread before. But the experienced cook looks at the dough, touches it and then remembers the time when they made bread on a humid day and the same thing happened. The experienced cook adds a little more flour and adjusts the amount of salt and yeast in the recipe so that the bread will rise.

Experts in nursing practice differently than new nurses or novices. This is important when discussing evidence based practice and clinical decision making. Novices and experts use information differently. Their knowledge base related to clinical experience is vastly different. Patricia Benner, nurse theorist of the "novice to expert model" for nursing has written extensively on the subject.

Benner's model of nursing knowledge defines five stages of nursing expertise (Benner, Tanner, & Chesla, 1996). The first stage or novice stage is exemplified in the graduate nurse. The novice applies the "rules" she has been taught because she has no clinical experience to draw from in decision making. Advanced beginners are still very much guided by policy and procedure. They consider objective facts and start to use more sophisticated rules. The advanced beginner starts to recognize situational elements relating to the skill of nursing. The competent nurse reaches a point where she must learn to prioritize importance in a particular situation. The competent nurse creates new rules based on the understanding that there are so many unique situations that one cannot possibly have a rule for each situation. The competent nurse begins to learn to live with the ambiguity of patient care. Benner says that the competent nurse begins to feel great responsibility for his actions. Whereas the novice and advanced beginner cannot make mistakes if they follow the rules (if a problem occurs it is the fault of the rule maker/teacher), the competent nurse has an "increased sense of urgency and responsibility for her knowledge of the patient" (p. 97). Benner states that the novice and advanced beginner take a "rule-following stance" that distances the nurse from the situation. A proficient nurse, however, demonstrates "increased perceptual accuracy and responsiveness to the particular situation" and an ability for "a perceptual grasp of qualitative distinctions [between patients], which can only be acquired by seeing and contrasting many similar and distinct clinical situations as they evolve over time" (p. 114). The response of the proficient nurse is not automatic; she must still think about what to do. The expert nurse's actions "reflect an attunement to the situation that allows responses to be shaped by a watchful reading of the patient's responses without recourse to conscious deliberation" (p. 143). Expert nurses use intuition as well as clinical expertise and knowledge in decision making. Expert nurses have a deep understanding of the "big picture." They exhibit an ability to integrate knowledge.

Integrative nursing takes experience and expertise. Integration as a highly developed professional ability can be a goal for all nurses, from novice to expert. So often the novice nurse is inundated with rules, policies, and requests for outcomes or evidence. The newly educated nurse is not presented with the big picture. When interacting with a more experienced nurse the novice may ask the question, "Where is your evidence?" or "How do you know?" This can alienate the expert nurse who should, by all accounts, be mentoring the novice. Sometimes the expert might "know" according to the literature, but sometimes the answer is related to an intuitive sense and expertise. Young nurses must be prepared to respect all the ways of knowing demonstrated by their mentors in providing nursing care.

It is of utmost importance that professional nursing experts not be pushed out of practice by the new attention to evidence-based practice (EBM) and outcomes research. Watching an expert nurse in action is a beautiful experience. The grace and wisdom they exude is remarkable. Nurse educators, in their zeal to impart the best of EBM, might consider the benefits of teaching Benner's model along with EBM so as to appropriately *frame* the process of *knowing in nursing* as drawing upon many sources, including research evidence *and* nurses' clinical expertise. This instills respect for those that have laid down, and often beaten down, the professional path.

Telling the Story

As is demonstrated in the narratives of the ten nurses in Chapter 4, nurses have a wealth of knowledge, experience, and expertise when it comes to demonstrating care. The nurses I spoke with told their stories with joy and humility. Each and every one had experienced being a part of changing the lives of their patients. Many memories were made. Each story of the ten nurses was unique because the nurses and their patients were unique. Nurses help others by telling their stories. Benner writes, "The oral tradition is effective in setting up salient memories. Stories are more memorable than lists of warnings that must be memorized out of context. Narrative memory sets up identification with the storyteller, creates an emotional response that causes the warning to become salient. Narratives also create sensibilities and imagination that enhance the clinician's perceptions and responses" (Benner et al., 1996, p. 208).

Benner is correct that memories of both patients and experiences are critical to developing nursing expertise and building a repertoire of experience from which to draw upon in practice. The storytelling of experienced nurses is not only helpful to other nurses, but also storytelling is a caring modality to use with patients. Storytelling is helpful in building rapport with patients. Patients love to tell *their* stories. They love to be listened to. Nurses can create relationship "bonds," as strong as the hydrogen bonds of DNA, by asking to hear their patients' stories. Nurses can gain insight into the needs and goals of the patient as they emerge from the hidden fabric of a tale.

I once took over care for a supposedly comatose patient whose wife was irate that the nursing staff had not been taking care of her husband. A part of me wanted to run away from the woman because I knew that I was going to have to listen to a lot of anger that I did not cause. I decided to be proactive and take some time to sit with this woman and listen to her "story." She did begin by talking about her anger toward the nursing staff for what she perceived as their inattention to her husband's needs. She talked about her responsibility to speak for him because he could not speak for himself. As I observed this woman's interaction with her husband, it was clear that she had a profound love for him. Although the patient was supposed to be comatose, he responded to her with hand gestures as she spoke with me. He had never done this with the nursing staff. The wife became calm and apologetic as I listened to her concerns and love for her husband. I told her that I could see how much she loved him.

As she relaxed, she explained that many of her husband's hand gestures were "conducting." Her husband had been a successful concert pianist his whole life. This was why she had been so concerned about preventing the contractures of his hands and had requested fewer finger pricks for blood sugar testing. For many years, her role in life had been the protector of her husband's hands. As she briefly told me the story of her husband's career, he became animated in the bed, swirling his arms as best he could. My semicomatose patient even opened his eyes a little. I'll never forget the story she told or that experience. The storytelling intervention opened the door to reasoning with the wife about my abilities and limitations in caring for her husband. Expertise in caring is given and received through the experience of listening and telling stories. Expertise in nursing is exemplified in the ability to make decisions with patients by accessing the memories of previous experiences as a guide to the present situation.

CLINICAL DECISION MAKING

As we listen to the stories of our patients, we realize even more the importance of tailoring our care to the individual patient. Nurses historically have valued the individual. Nurses know very well the uncertainty that comes with rejecting a "cookbook" approach to nursing care. There are many biomedical skills we perform that are best done a particular way for all patients. But as with the IV example, the modalities chosen to express caring, compassion, and, yes, even love, are often different for each and every patient. Perhaps the uncertainty or ambiguity of the non-cookbook approach frightens some nurses. The "intractable source of uncertainty is the individuality of the patient . . . the more important the knowledge required by the decision, the less tolerable is the uncertainty" (Cassell, 1993, p. 36). Cookbook approaches are not only done with biomedical skills. Often nurses who have experience and knowledge of a particular caring modality will use the modality with each patient without regarding the individual needs of a given patient.

In clinical decision making, nurses who develop a repertoire of caring modalities must understand the importance of keen observation and of assessing the *appropriateness* of the modality in the care of the individual patient. The integrative nurse must make all decisions regarding caring modalities with the consent and input of the patient or the family. The nurse thinks through how the caring modality used with a patient will enhance the healing ability of the patient and provide support for the patient who is trying to achieve greater balance.

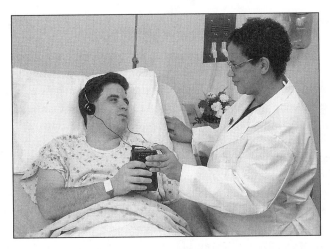

Music is the chosen caring modality

For example, nurses who have studied professional massage do not always give every patient a massage. Nurses who have skills and knowledge in massage bring to the healing relationship the opportunity for the patient to *choose* having massage. In their interactions with patients, experienced nurses come to depend upon the choices of patients. "The finding that experienced and skilled nurses described situations of different degrees of depth of contact with patients to whom caring was said to make a difference, can be expressed in the phrase, 'it depends on the situation how I act.' The fact that the nurses stressed the importance of the situation at hand indicates that they reason as experts or proficient nurses" (Astrom, Norberg, & Hallberg, 1995, p. 192). Nurses' provision of any caring modality is dependent upon the timing and the appropriateness of the intervention for the patient.

The integrative nurse, after assessing the unique patient situation, then looks at the skills of the patient in caring for himself. The nurse also looks at ways she might be helpful in caring for the patient. There are hundreds of caring modalities. Nurses cannot learn them all, and this really isn't the goal. The goal is to create and maintain a healing relationship, the therapeutic use of self in relation with the patient. What the nurse brings to that relationship as far as *what* caring modalities to use in practice is the nurse's *choice. How* the nurse uses those modalities in practice depends on the nurse's professional *creativity.*

CREATIVITY AND CHOICE

Creativity in nursing is exemplified by the nurse's ability to adapt any caring modality to the unique needs of the patient. I often think of my rural nursing days and how the simple, even rustic, environment in which we practiced forced us to "get creative" in meeting the needs of the patients. Helping people in chronic pain is one example. I took care of a patient one weekend who was not getting relief from her prescribed pain medication. It was the weekend and no pharmacies were open. The patient and I decided that she would meditate and take hot baths along with the pain medication to help her maintain a certain level of comfort until she could get a stronger medication on Monday morning. I provided listening support for her as well.

Another example of choosing a caring modality in my own practice is the use of dance and movement with children, in particular infants and their parents. Dance therapy is considered a complementary therapy now, but in the 1970s, when I studied at New York University, there were no "alternative and complementary therapies" per se. Dance itself, and more recently since the early 1900s movement analysis and dance therapy, has been used in healing practices in many countries throughout the world. In working with children, I have found my education and experience in the field of dance to be invaluable in sharpening my observation skills, increasing my ability to communicate with nonverbal children, and in understanding my own nonverbal communication with patients.

I have integrated my love of dance and movement into my work as a nurse. As a nurse, I am fascinated by human behavior and the way people move or don't move. Although I may not structure a dance therapy session with a patient per se, I still *integrate* my knowledge and practice of dance and movement in my work with children. For example, I often work with mothers and babies who are adapting to each other's bodies in the process of breast-feeding. Breast-feeding is an intimate "dance" that occurs between mother and infant. I often assist mothers to harmonize the flow of movements between themselves and their infants. I integrate the science of movement analysis and therapy (which includes understanding effort, as discussed in Chapter 3) with my nurse's understanding of promoting lactation to help the infant-mother feeding relationship.

Just as I have used my understanding of the science and art of movement and dance in building healing relationships with patients, so have nurses skilled in other areas that are complementary to fundamental nursing practices used their talents. The nurse who enjoys finding new ways of helping patients can allow herself to creatively compose an entire repertoire of modalities from which to draw upon in any healing relationship.

Creativity takes courage. It also takes trust and peace. When nurses trust themselves and their patients, creative thoughts can flow. When nurses trust the healing relationship and the creativity in problem solving and allowing for healing to occur, there is often an opportunity to relax and experience a greater sense of peace. This is not always easy, and nurses often feel somewhat anxious when they allow themselves to be creative in patient care. Rollo May speaks of the anxiety experienced during the creative process as being part of the "breakthrough" of insight leading to new ideas. May writes, "The breakthrough carries with it also an element of anxiety. For it not only broke down my previous hypothesis, it shook my self-world relationship. At such a time I find myself having to seek a new foundation, the existence of which I as yet don't know. This is the source of the anxious feeling that comes at the moment of the breakthrough; it is not possible that there be a genuinely new idea without this shakeup occurring to some degree" (1994, p. 60). Having an insight and implementing that insight is creative and takes courage. Nurses have a history of exemplifying both creativity and a pioneering spirit. Nurses know the importance of the creative process as being a source of breakthroughs and new knowledge. Nursing practice is reenergized by new knowledge and new ideas.

New ideas come forth from the experience of nurses. Nurses have insights all the time in their experiences with patients. Insight is what keeps the profession *alive.* May defines insight as a "state of heightened consciousness" (1994, p. 61). He writes that insights *"never come hit or miss, but in accordance with a pattern of which one essential element is our own commitment* . . . the insight is born from unconscious levels exactly in the areas in which we are most intensively consciously committed" (pp. 61, 62).

Nurses who practice from an integrative perspective must be committed to the healing relationship, meeting the needs of the patient and providing care. The caring modalities the nurse uses in practice are instruments that help him realize these commitments. Often the commitment will bring forth insight. The greater the intensity of the commitment, the greater the need for allowing insight to be present in the relationship. In the case of nursing, the patient as well as the nurse can bring forth the insight. The observant nurse can tell when an "insight of healing" has emerged from the healing relationship. Often the use of an appropriate caring modality will place the patient or nurse in the position of being able to receive healing insight, that "ah-ha" moment experienced by the patient with the half-paralyzed esophagus (Chapter 10).

Choosing to use a caring modality such as massage, therapeutic touch, herbal tea, communication, hydrotherapies, electromagnetic therapies, or energy therapy with patients takes courage and understanding. The nurse who decides to scientifically and artistically explore the use of caring modalities in providing patient care can be reassured that experiencing anxiety is a *normal* part of the creative process.

The creative process must continue for the growth of nursing as a caring profession. For too long, nurses have focused much of their time and energy on the development of biomedical nursing science. We have much to be proud of. As we begin a new millennium, nurses must return to their fundamental caring skills, which are historically significant and carry a rich and well-defined legacy. Embracing the creative process in our profession means encouraging freedom of choice, intuition as well as knowledge, and the opportunity to integrate all that we are individually, as well as all that we are as a profession of scientists and artists.

The evolution of science and art are dependent on each other. One cannot occur without the other. Creativity is as important to science as it is to art. Embracing creativity allows nurses the opportunity to explore the deeper dimensions of the health and healing experience of their patients and themselves. Nurses in all specialties, including the highly technical areas, and even more so perhaps in the highly technical specialties, need to be encouraged to use their creative abilities. Nurses must deal with the blocks to their creativity from within and without or we may be in danger of losing more than the art of nursing; we may risk losing the science of nursing as well. "To the extent that we lose this free, original creativity of the spirit as it is exemplified in poetry and music and art, we shall also lose our scientific creativity. I am proposing that creativity . . . is not only important for art and poetry and music; but is essential in the long run also for our science. To shrink from the anxiety this entails, and block off the threatening new insights and forms this engenders, is not only to render our society banal and progressively more empty, but also to cut off as well the headwaters in the rough and rocky mountains of the stream that later becomes the river of creativity in our science" (May, 1994, pp. 69–72).

Caring modalities offer the opportunity for creativity. They are the tools or instruments of the nurse's art and science. Nurses must choose caring modalities that uphold and enhance their commitment to patient care and respect that the choices of caring modalities are personal and may be different for each nurse. In the art world, some people are better painters than musicians, and therefore they choose the brush rather than a violin. Both can create beautiful art. Nurses have many caring modalities from which to choose. None is more important than another; all *art* that comes from a commitment of the *heart* has its place in patient care.

Conclusion

As nurses continue to grow and gain confidence in practice, they will identify their area of expertise in providing care that is both science- and art-based. It is to the experts in nursing that others can look for inspiration to take the profession to new heights and new adventures. One student nurse writes of the inspiring act of a nurse leader, "I am looking forward towards a time of post-academic nursing practice, when we take for granted the notion that excellence is grounded in research and we have moved on to embrace the qualities of love and intuition that currently make us squiggle with embarrassment. I am convinced that it is the need to give love, even more than to be loved, which brings many people into nursing. Why do we find it so difficult to talk about?" (Allen, 1992, p. 24). Perhaps, if it is difficult to talk about, nurses can place more attention on *demonstrating* love and care instead.

References

Allen, C. (1992). Ode to joy. *Nursing Times, 88* (10), 24.

Astrom, G., Norberg, A., Hallberg, I., & Jansson, L. (1993). Experienced and skilled nurses' narratives of situations where caring action made a difference to the patient. *Scholarly Inquiry for Nursing Practice: An International Journal, 7* (3), 183–193.

Benner, P., Tanner, C., & Chesla, C. (1996). *Expertise in nursing practice.* New York: Springer Publishing Co.

Cassell, E. J. (1993). The sorcerer's broom: Medicine's rampant technology. *Hastings Center Report, 23* (6), 32–39.

May, R. (1994). *The courage to create.* New York: W.W. Norton.

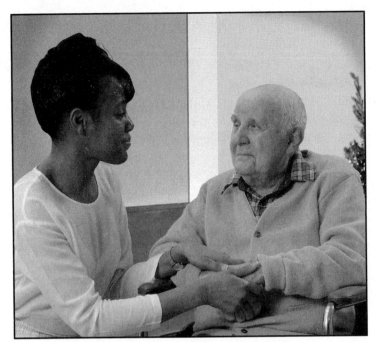

Communication through touch

If we did all the things we are capable of doing,

we would literally astound ourselves.

—THOMAS EDISON

CHAPTER 14

The Growth of a Caring Profession

A s we begin a new millennium, nurses will continue to find new ways of integrating biomedical skills with the historical foundation of nursing practice in the science and art of caring. Integration can be an easier process of change than one in which an old way of doing things is replaced with a new way. Old ways are so familiar and comfortable and often make people happy. It is human nature to hold on to that which is comfortable and familiar. New ways, no matter how beneficial they may potentially be, are often perceived as uncomfortable and threatening. Creating change both personally and professionally by throwing out "the old" and replacing it with "the new" can leave some people feeling uneasy. The *integration* of old and new when trying to create change is often better received and gives people the opportunity to feel good about growth.

I've heard administrators in health care talk about "letting nurses go" who don't want to change and work with new ways of providing health care. Is this really the answer for the healthy growth of a *caring* profession? This method sounds very much like one of the ways of dealing with a problem in the biomedical model—if there is a problem, just surgically remove it. There are integrated approaches to change, growth, and balance of power.

The Powers That Be

Just as the upward curve of each helix in the healing relationship model winds its way around its solid axis, nurses in relationship continue to define and redefine professional values, healing philosophies, and scope of practice around the "axis" of caring. Although we all might agree that caring is the foundation of what we do as nurses, how caring is demonstrated is often very different from nurse to nurse, town to town, and country to country. So many variables influence the choices nurses make in how they will demonstrate caring. The individual application of a caring modality with the unique patient is rarely the same. Some nurses are comfortable with variation between the way their colleagues provide care and some are not. How often has it been said by one nurse to another, "That's not the way *we* do it here." As nursing grows as a caring profession, and nurses take more personal responsibility for the development of their own practices, it is more and more apparent that there will be greater need for tolerance and appreciation of individual differences expressed as creativity in the art and science of nursing.

Nurses want and need to be creative in their work. Inherent in the creative process is the ability to keep the joy of commitment to patient care alive. One nurse seeking control over another's practice is the very antithesis of the creation of an environment that values creativity and individual professionalism and commitment. Nurses have often been trained in facilities that do not necessarily foster individual creativity and accountability. Because of this history, it is understandable why some nurses balk at the concept of being responsible for creatively planning care for a patient. Physicians direct patient care. Nurses can direct patient care *with* the patient. The "powers that be" are represented in the many faces and voices of those who would keep nurses in the old mold of subservience and dependence. The "powers that be" are also represented in the habitual thought patterns of some nurses who wait in the comfort zone of being told how, when, and where to practice caring rather than taking the risk and responsibility of making independent decisions. This is not to say that every nurse, novice to expert, must become a leader. There are some nurses who do not and will never feel comfortable leading their own practice. But those who do want to "fly," as did Jonathan Livingston Seagull, must be supported. Diversity in nursing practice must be supported for the sake of the diverse population we serve.

As nurses find ways to allow for greater creativity to emerge in their own practices, there also must be a greater awareness of how nurses and the entire health team collaborate for the benefit of the patient. The ways nurses work together may change. With greater sense of individuality in practice comes greater responsibility and the necessity to work in harmony with other practitioners as well as with patients. It's like the double helix, self in relation again. Nurses have the skills to collaborate with others. A fully integrative model of patient care suggests a need for practitioners who genuinely value collaboration. To practice integrative nursing and to be able to collaborate with patients and other practitioners, the team must accept and find value in understanding professional and individual differences as well as similarities.

I learned growing up in the theatre that everyone involved in a production, with all of their similarities and differences, has something to give. Although everyone has their own way of doing things, there is a process of sharing, and even compromise, among a group of creative professionals that allows for the realization of the goals of performance—pleasing an audience. Perhaps nurses in the new millennium will gain insight into the collaborative process by observing the world of art. Take the symphony, for example. As an audience sits listening to the music of an incredible composer, such as Ludwig van Beethoven, they experience every sound, every instrument, and every musician. Some musicians play constantly, the violinists. Some play rarely, the percussionist playing the cymbals. One musician is not more important than another.

I had been taught this as a dancer, that none in the theatre was any more important than another. I learned that if the lighting master missed his cue I would be standing on the stage in the dark. I learned if I missed a cue my partner would look pretty silly on stage in front of the audience. Although each dancer was responsible for his performance there was a sense of interdependence on each other for the performance as a whole to be a success. It is the same when listening to Beethoven. Every instrument is important and unique. The conductor and the musicians all know very well the importance of each instrument and musician to the arrangement of beautiful music. Perhaps some nurses don't get a chance to experience their importance in the

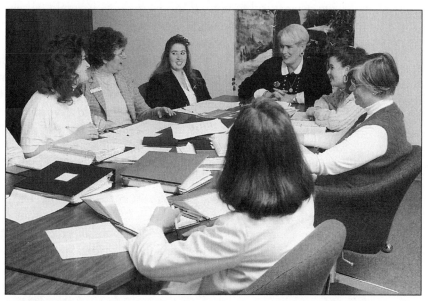

Collaboration

"musical score" of health care. This may be because their "performance" is often with an individual patient and not with a whole "audience" of patients. But nevertheless, nurses would surely benefit from the opportunity of knowing their importance to the greater "design" or "arrangement" in health care.

THE SYMPHONY METAPHOR

Nurses who have felt insignificant in a large health care organization can probably relate to this story. The story takes place in a managed care company in which the president has a ticket to a performance of Schubert's Unfinished Symphony. Because the president was unable to go to the symphony, she gave her ticket to one of her managed care reviewers. The next morning she asked him how he liked the symphony and he sent her a memo saying:

1. For a considerable period the oboe players had nothing to do. Their numbers should be reduced and their work spread over the whole orchestra, thus avoiding peaks of inactivity.
2. All twelve violins were playing identical notes. This seems like unnecessary duplication and the staff of this section should be drastically cut. If a large volume of sound is really required, this could be obtained through the use of an amplifier.
3. Much effort was involved in playing the sixteenth notes. This seems an excessive refinement. It is recommended that all notes should be rounded up to the nearest eighth note. If this were done, it would be possible to use paraprofessionals instead of experienced musicians.
4. No useful purpose is served by repeating with the horns the passage that has already been handled by the strings. If such redundant passages were eliminated, the concert could be reduced from two hours to twenty minutes.
5. This symphony has two movements. If Schubert didn't achieve his goals by the end of the first movement, then he should have stopped there. The second movement is unnecessary and should be cut. In light of the above, one can only conclude that had Schubert given attention to these matters, he probably would have had time to finish his symphony.

This story demonstrates the environment nurses often practice in on a daily basis. The art, or ability to be creative, in practice is often driven out from professional nursing by the "powers that be," with American managed care companies being just one example. It is because of this pressure that many nurses no longer realize that their work is important. They no longer realize that *they* are important. Many nurses lack the sense of their *unique gift* to the healing and health care of others.

Some never seem to get the opportunity to discover the "sense of the unique gift" in nursing school either. Education comes from the word *educare,* meaning to bring forth. Do nurses get the chance to bring forth their special gifts of healing and caring in school as they memorize all the details of nursing work they need to know to be safe and efficient in the clinical setting? According to the retired nurses I've spoken to, there is less of a focus on the creative and unique aspect of care today than there used to be. This lack of understanding of the unique gift carries over to the practice setting as well. If the same nurses who do not have a sense of the unique gift of each nurse become administrators or educators, they may feel more comfortable advocating the cookbook approach to nursing.

Then the struggle begins. Nurses are often forced to choose between being the type of nurse who plays by "the rules," with the emphasis on what can be called the duties of nursing, and being the type of nurse who experiments and creates new ways of caring as she gives full recognition to the unique qualities of the patient and herself. Nurses can decide to choose to integrate rather than separate. Nurses can respect rules, duties, and collaborative practice *and* be creative and unique. Integrative nursing is meant to be a model of harmony and balance just like the symphony. In the symphony, each instrument has a beauty all its own, and when the instruments are played together, harmonious music results. Each nurse has her own beauty and gift for caring to offer to the health care team.

In 1991, an article was published in *Nursing Administration Quarterly* that discussed the importance of a "clear nursing identity." "One of the greatest potential difficulties for the nursing profession as health care becomes more decentralized is the fragmentation of the nursing service and the loss of a clear nursing identity and control over nursing practice. Nursing will unquestionably increase in value to the system. Nurses can fit almost any service arrangement and provide a valuable service. However, what will be in place to ensure that the profession's values, roles, and integrity get affirmed and reinforced in the individual nurse when delivery models become increasingly dissimilar?" (Porter-O'Grady, 1991, p. 4).

Nursing fundamentals or caring modalities carry the identity that is nursing. Nurses who value fundamentals as part of professional nursing practice must negotiate services in their organizations that include the caring modalities that have been a part of nursing's historical tradition. When nurses demonstrate the importance of an integrative practice that includes caring modalities to organizational leadership, nurses will be acting to preserve nursing identity, the foundation upon which scientific and artistic creativity can emerge. There is often a lack of clarity in organizations about nurses' roles. "There is a tendency to revise roles and responsibilities based on what the institution perceives versus what the professional standards and values support. Nurses are professionals first and employees of an institution second" (Koerner, Bunkers, & Nelson, 1991, p. 16). Nurses must negotiate a service delivery model that reflects their values of developing healing relationships and providing caring modalities.

Nurses, as professionals, need to claim their history with the caring modalities now being labeled "complementary and alternative *medicine*" and protect their right

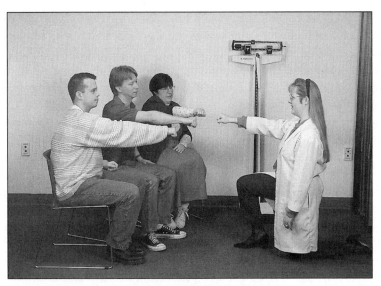

Nurses demonstrating progressive muscle relaxation

to choose these modalities as part of nursing practice and nursing identity. Nurses must protect their rights to determine the practice of their profession. The thought that any biomedical establishment would claim rights to controlling the practice of complementary therapies in any country is a threat to health practices freedom. Benjamin Rush, Surgeon General of the Continental Army of the United States and signer of the Declaration of Independence is quoted as saying, "The Constitution of this Republic should make special provision for Medical Freedom as well as Religious Freedom. . . . To restrict the art of healing to one class of men and deny equal privileges to others will constitute the Bastille of medical science" (as qtd. in Dossey & Swyers, 1992).

Nurses represent patient care. Nurses advocate for patient rights and the freedom to choose how, when, and where a healing relationship is begun and what type of modalities will be used. The future of nursing care depends upon the preservation of health freedom and the patient and caregiver's freedom to choose.

Using the symphony metaphor once more, as nurses continue to grow as a caring profession, nurses must continue to strive to be "on the same sheet of music" professionally and have a recognized "conductor" to guide the process. Perhaps the "same sheet of music" is the commitment to creating evolving, healing relationships with patients and the encouragement of creativity in discovering and researching old and new ways of demonstrating care. Perhaps the "conductor" of the symphony of caregivers in nursing is "nature" itself, which Florence Nightingale defined as the true healer.

Suffering or Self-care

Before a symphony begins, the musicians randomly enter the stage, dressed in black and white. They do not sit down in their chairs, open their music, and begin to play the music scheduled for the evening's performance. They warm up first. In dance theatre, we do the same. Before any performance, I have a ritual. I get to the theatre two hours before the performance and spend up to an hour warming up my body by stretching. I drink a cup of tea, do any last minute preparation of my costume and put on my makeup. I then prepare mentally and spiritually, in my own way, for dancing in harmony with the music, with other performers, and with the audience for whom I have never performed. In the dance world, this process is called *centering*. In the music world, it is called *tuning up*. Basically, it's all the same thing; it's a process of readying oneself, taking care of one's *self* first so that others can be served.

Nurses have taught others the process of self-care for decades. Dorothea Orem even developed a model called the self-care model (Orem, 1991). Yet, I often wonder how many nurses take the time and space to take care of themselves, the very least of which is to prepare for their daily work with patients. Jean Watson writes, "We have to treat ourselves with gentleness and dignity before we can respect and care for others with gentleness and dignity" (Watson, 1988, p. 33). Part of that expression of respect for self lies in the self-care we do before and after patient care. Nurses as human beings are in need of healing just as their patients are. It is by acknowledging this humanness to ourselves that we affirm our need for self-care, tuning up, and centering. Nurses are the bearers of the cup of cool water to many, but the cup that continually pours ultimately runs dry. The cup must straighten up (centering), ask to be filled (tune up), and *be* filled (self-care) before it can pour forth again. This flow or process of pouring forth and being filled over and over again, is a dance of service to life. Like the curves of the helix, the nurse becomes more adept at learning with each opportunity for renewal and pouring forth, how to maintain her physical, mental, and spiritual strength and balance while engaging every day those whose lives are full of suffering.

Many of the environments nurses work in are not very nurturing and healing for the nurses or the patients. For this reason, "caring for caregivers" is important. Nurses need caring because they enter intimate relationships with patients in which intense emotions can be experienced. Much of nurses' work involves strong emotions of grief, loss, sadness, depression, and anxiety. One study by Menzies Lyth (1959) showed that "on the basis of intensive interviews with nursing personnel a lack of support and reassurance can be particularly painful for some nurses who must not only observe the caring concern extended to patients, but are also required to deliver such care themselves. A significant number of nurses . . . perceive the hospital as an organization particularly well equipped to deal with dependency needs, kind and supportive, and they expect to have the privilege of being very dependent themselves. As a result of these unaccommodated and unresolved dependency needs, nurses frequently experience envy towards the recipients of the care which they themselves desire" (as cited in Holden, 1991, p. 894). It is quite normal that a nurse who is caring for others would want to be cared for as well when she is needy or suffering. Unfortunately, nurses come to realize that although individuals within an organization might care for them, the "organizations" per se are not capable of caring for them. More important is the question of whether or not the nurse is aware of when she is needy and suffering and whether those needs ever get met.

Nurses must encourage themselves to "tune" into their own needs and times of suffering. They must have a ritual time, like the artist before a performance, when they "center" themselves and make sure that their "instruments" are ready to "play," or serve others. So how does a nurse know that she has a need or is suffering? Nurses often do not recognize the intensity and importance of the unseen emotional labor of nursing practice and how it can take its toll on the ability to serve others. A nurse might be sitting with a patient, listening intently and then say, "Well, I have to go do some work now." If nurses do not view the emotional work they do with patients in a healing relationship as *real work,* and that their "cup" is almost empty, then how will they know when they need to fill the cup again? Not valuing one's work and not paying attention to one's own needs for healing can ultimately be experienced by the body and the spirit as self-torture.

Judy Tatelbaum writes in her book, *You Don't Have to Suffer,* "We are our own worst enemy whenever we indulge in what Fritz Perls called 'self tortures.' Coping by indulging in destructive thinking processes, such as obsessive thinking, complaining, worry, regret, and guilt, can consume us and make us feel powerless to control our lives. Self-torturing behaviors are usually so automatic that we may not have known until now that they deplete our energy and impede our handling of our lives. The purpose in uncovering these behaviors is to free us to choose, if we wish, to let them go and to find more satisfying ways of dealing with life" (1989, pp. 67–68). Embracing the work they have done as being truly meaningful and healing allows nurses to be better able to treat themselves and others with gentleness and dignity. The self-torture ends and the "music" can begin.

No matter how seemingly insignificant nursing might be to some, it is not insignificant to nurses and their patients. Provision of nursing care can be a wondrous, energizing, and healing experience. For some nurses like Florence Nightingale, the work is the fulfillment of a calling of the soul. Entering into the healing process, the healing relationship with a patient takes courage and love. The nurse must be aware of the care of his own needs as much as the needs of others. It is truly a process, a flow between knowing when to pour forth and when to refill the cup. This calling is not for everyone, but it is for nurses.

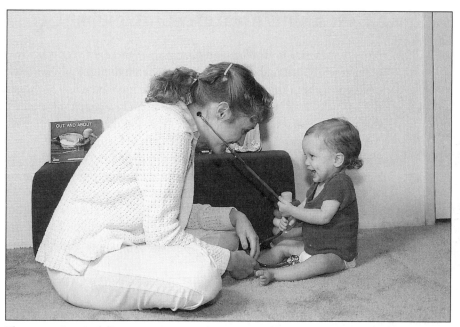

Play as a caring modality

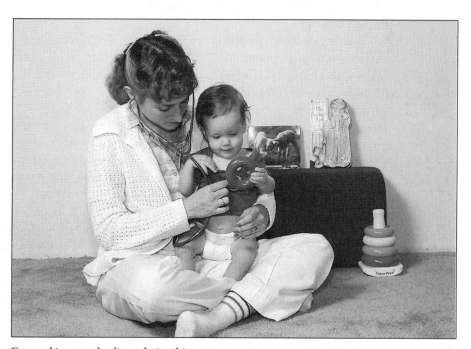

Engaged in a new healing relationship

Growing a New Skin: Integrative Integument

Nursing practice is growing and changing, sometimes very quickly. Sometimes it may seem easier to just make a change rather than to figure out ways to hold onto what has been good about the past. I think of my kitchen where it is always easier to throw out the leftovers than try to find a way to use them in a recipe the next day. I am not saying that all that nurses have done in the past should be integrated into practice today. Maybe there are some things better left to the history books. As with the example of nurses' caring modalities, now called complementary therapies, there may be some nursing practices that should be reexplored. Integration can mean pulling together all that has been and is meaningful into a new form. This new form consists of a strong foundation or structure from the past, the freshness of the present, and the tremendous opportunity and anticipation of the future. The new form has new definition or boundaries that contain the matrix of past, present, and future within it. Integrative nursing is a new form or matrix.

The growth process of taking on the new form of integrative nursing practice is much like the growth of new skin. The skin is what defines a person in space; it provides form. The skin is a boundary that defines the relationship between the self and the environment. The process of growing new skin can be seen as redefining one's boundaries. The process is also significant in what it can teach us as we generalize the concept of growing new physical skin to the growth of the new "skin" of integrative nursing practice.

I use the example of the skin because it is a miraculous organ in its ability to regenerate while maintaining the integrity of being. The skin serves as a constant reminder of the body's natural life force and energy capable of rejuvenation. When a body grows new skin, some old skin cells slough off and new cells replace the old. There is no time when one area of the body is left raw and open while new skin is being formed. The integrity of the integument is maintained during the process of growth. It is a continual process of which the person is usually unconscious unless there is some insult or injury to the skin. Although there is considerable change, there is no pain. As with the growth of new skin, integrative nursing can be rejuvenating. The following principles for integration are based upon lessons from human skin:

1. All growth must maintain the boundary and integrity of the individual. When old skin sloughs off there is always new skin to replace it. When nurses make changes, individually or professionally, be aware of the process. Is the new "skin" in place? Does the old skin really need to come off, now or ever? Can the old and new "skin" overlap or integrate in any way? For example, seek ways to *add* to your observation skills and your repertoire of biomedical and caring modalities, perhaps even by learning a type of complementary therapy and finding ways to creatively integrate the new caring modality into your practice.

2. Some surface cells may change and die but the underlying integument or foundation remains the same so that ongoing growth can continue. Nurses who know what they value in regards to patient care have a strong foundation for "surface" changes to occur professionally and personally. Without a strong foundation in the care of patients, new modalities and practice models will be difficult to evaluate and utilize.

3. The environment affects the skin and sometimes changes it, such as changes in skin pigment related to exposure to the sun. Too much exposure to certain environmental elements can be toxic and detrimental to growth. The skin represents a boundary both physical and psychological. Nurses who know who they are and what they are about communicate strong boundaries to those they encounter in their environment. Nurses interact continually with people who may not understand the nature of the nursing profession or its work. Nurses need to be aware when they have identified too much with the people and environments in which they work and too little with their inner calling and education as a professional nurse. It takes keen observation to know when the "exposure" is damaging the boundary.

4. The skin must be nourished from the inside as well as the outside to remain healthy. It is not sufficient to use Band-Aids and creams to heal wounds or maintain normal skin growth and function. Healthy skin depends very much on a healthy diet and adequate hydration with water as well. Nurses do not only alleviate symptoms with Band-Aids and creams; they use a holistic approach to health care and can continue to grow in the exploration of new ways of providing a holistic blend of biomedical and caring modalities.

5. Just as all skin cells know (i.e., are coded with DNA) how to regenerate, all nurses must be educated in the care of self-regeneration and centering. Nurses must be able to care for their bodies, to deal with debilitating stress through relaxation, meditation, exercise, and create a healing environment for self; to get enough rest; drink pure water, and eat the foods that charge one's battery and give pleasure; to nurture oneself with social and spiritual relationships and experiences; and to get the health care that is needed.

6. There are many different cultures of peoples with very different skin tones. Although the pigment underneath may be different, all human skin has the same mission—to protect internal organs and define the person in space. Although there are many ways of providing nursing care, culture to culture, and individual nurse to individual nurse, underneath it all, our mission is the same—to create evolving, healing relationships with others in which caring is *demonstrated*.

Many portend that the new millennium will bring considerable change to all areas of life including the way we heal. Growth is inevitable now as it has always been. It is not a question of whether or not growth will occur but how it will occur. Will the growth of the caring profession of nursing be like the wild cell growth of a skin melanoma or perhaps just a gentle wrinkling over time as wisdom, experience, and happiness leave their mark on the "skins" of the nurses who embrace their path as healers and comforters to humankind? The decision is ours individually and collectively. There is always a choice.

Conclusion

The practice of integrative nursing embraces change as a constant—change as a process of adding to and rearranging, as well as taking away. Change can be big or it can be small. All change must occur within a structure. The structure is the history and experiences of many expert nurses. It is every nurse's and every patient's health beliefs. It is sociocultural norms regarding healing and health care. Integrative nursing invites nurses to be all that they are in practice. Nurses do not have to make radical changes to familiar structures to be able to provide the kind of care and healing they would want to receive if they were ill. Structure exists to provide support for change and growth. It is not meant to be a deterrent or a limit to change, growth, or creativity.

Nursing is a vital healing art and science. Nurses scientifically experiment and artistically create in their interactions with patients as they attune through touch, create healing environments, nurture with nutritious food, connect through various forms of communication, and enliven with attention to energy. The freedom to experiment and create is expressed in the healing relationship, the focus of patient care.

Through involvement with others in healing relationships, nurses learn that it is often the experience of a physical or emotional imbalance or illness that brings people to a place in their lives where they explore their reason for being, their beliefs about health and life, and their relationships to others and the environment. Nurses are a witness to this process and are able to help patients be gentle with themselves during this time of reflection and self-concern.

Nurses are compassionate caregivers who create healing environments where patients can get to know themselves. As patients learn more about their own nature and their health and illness experiences, they can learn to love who they are. People who are able to love themselves, especially when they are ill and vulnerable, are better able to love others as themselves. They are also better able to care for or "do unto others" as they would have others do unto them—fulfilling the golden rule. The world needs more compassion. Nurses have the skills and the means to demonstrate those skills of compassion, caring, and love that have developed over centuries of being present at the right moment to enter into a relationship with someone in need of healing. As we go about our work with "simplicity and singleness of heart" as Florence Nightingale said (1957, p. 76), we are examples of compassion and love. And ultimately this is the goal of nursing care: to be an example of love, to love others as ourselves, and to love ourselves enough to know at every level of our being that we, too, are worthy of the love and caring that emerge from the very heart of the healing relationship.

References

Dossey, L., & Swyers, J. (1992). *Alternative medicine: Expanding medical horizons.* A report to the National Institute of Health on Alternative Medical Systems and Practices in the United States. (pp. xxxviii–xlviii). Washington, D.C.: Government Printing Office.

Holden, R. (1991). An analysis of caring: attributions, contributions and resolutions. *Journal of Advanced Nursing, 16,* 893–898.

Koerner, J. G., Bunkers, S. S., & Nelson, J. (1991). Change: A professional challenge. *Nursing Administration Quarterly, 16* (1), 15–21.

Menzies Lyth, I.E.P. (1959). The functioning of social systems as a defense against anxiety. In I. E. P. Menzies Lyth (Ed.), *Containing anxiety in institutions: Selected essays.* London: Free Association Books.

Nightingale, F. (1957). *Notes on nursing.* Philadelphia: J.B. Lippincott Co.

Orem, D. E. (1991). *Nursing: Concepts of practice* (4th ed.). St. Louis, MO: Mosby-Yearbook.

Porter-O'Grady, T. (1991). Changing realities for nursing: New models, new roles for nursing care delivery. *Nursing Administration Quarterly, 16* (1), 1–6.

Tatelbaum, J. (1989). *You don't have to suffer.* New York: Harper and Row.

Watson, J. (1988). *Nursing: Human science and human care.* New York: National League for Nursing.

List of Complementary and Alternative Medicine

This list of complementary and alternative medicine (CAM) was developed by the National Center for Complementary and Alternative Medicine (NCCAM)) at the National Institutes of Health in the United States (http://nccam.nih.gov/oam/).

Yoga
Internal Qi Gong
Tai Chi
Psychotherapy
Meditation
Imagery
Hypnosis
Biofeedback
Support Groups
Art Therapy
Music Therapy
Dance Therapy
Journaling
Humor
Body Psychotherapy
Confession
Nonlocality
Nontemporality

Soul Retrieval
Spiritual Healing
"Special" Healers
Caring-based Approaches (e.g., holistic nursing, pastoral care)
Intuitive Diagnosis
Placebo
Explanatory Models
Community-based Approaches (e.g., Alcoholics Anonymous, Native American "sweat" rituals)
Acupuncture
Herbal Formulas
Diet
External and Internal Qi Gong
Tai Chi
Massage and Manipulation (Tui Na)
Acupotomy

Native American Medicine
Ayurvedic Medicine
Unani-Tibbi, SIDDHI
Kampo Medicine
Traditional African Medicine
Traditional Aboriginal Medicine
Curanderismo
Central and South American Practices
Psychic Surgery
Homeopathy
Functional Medicine
Environmental Medicine
Radiesthesia, Psionic Medicine
Cayce-based Systems
Kneipp "classical"
Orthomolecular Medicine
Radionics
Anthroposophically-extended Medicine
Naturopathy
Electro-dermal Diagnostics
Medical Intuition
Chiriography
Functional Cellular Enzyme Measures
Panchakarma
Lifestyle Therapies
Health Promotion
Phytotherapy or Herbalism
Special Diet Therapies
   Pritikin
   Ornish
   McDougall
   Gerson
   Kelly-Gonzales
   Wigmore
   Livingston-Wheeler
   Atkins
   Diamond
   Vegetarian
   Fasting
   High Fiber
   Macrobiotic
   Mediterranean

   Paleolithic
   Asian
   Natural Hygiene
Orthomolecular Medicine
Apitherapy
Neural Therapy
Electrodiagnostics
Iridology
Bioresonance
MORA Device
Chiropractic Medicine
Massage and Body Work
Osteopathic Manipulative Therapy (OMT)
Cranial-Sacral OMT
Swedish Massage
Applied Kinesiology
Reflexology
Pilates Method
Polarity
Trager Body Work
Alexander Technique
Feldenkrais Technique
Acupressure
Rolfing
Hydrotherapy
Diathermy
Light and Color Therapies
Heat and Electrotherapies
Colonics
Alternate Nostril Breathing Techniques
Therapeutic Touch
Healing Science
Healing Touch
Natural Healing
SHEN
Mariue
Reiki
Huna
External Qi Gong
Biorelax
Bioelectromagnetics
Coley's Toxins

Antineoplastons
Cartilage
EDTA
Ozone
H_2O_2
Hyperbaric Oxygen
IAT
714X
MHT-68

Gallo Immunotherapy
Cone Therapy
Revici System
Enzyme Therapies
Cell Therapy
Enderlin Products
T/Tn Vaccine
Bee Pollen
Induced Remission Therapy

Resources for Further Learning: Touch Therapies/Bodywork

Reflexology Research:
Barbara and Kevin Kunz
Albuquerque, NM, USA
Phone: 1-505-344-9392
http://www.reflexology-research.com

Association of Reflexologists
London, England
Phone: 0870 5673320
http://www.reflexology.org
e-mail: aor@reflexology.org

International Institute of Reflexology
5650 First Avenue North
P.O. Box 12642
St. Petersburg, FL, USA 33733
Phone: 1-813-343-4811

Ersdal Zone Therapy Training
Christine Horvath
Academy of Dynamic Integrative Therapy
St. Paul, MN, USA
Phone: 1-800-250-4974

American Massage Therapy Association
Phone: 1-312-761-AMTA

Rolf Institute of Structural Integration
205 Canyon Blvd.
Boulder, CO, USA 80302
Phone: 1-800-530-8875

Hellerwork, Inc.
406 Berry St.
Mt. Shasta, CA, USA 96067
Phone: 1-800-392-3900 or 1-916-926-2500

The Trager Institute
33 Millwood St.
Mill Valley, CA, USA 94941
Phone: 1-415-388-2688
Fax: 1-415-388-2710

The Feldenkrais Guild
706 Ellsworth St.
P.O. Box 489
Albany, OR, USA 97321-0143
Phone: 1-800-775-2118 or 1-503-926-0981

Jin Shin Jyutsu, Inc.
8719 E. San Alberta
Scottsdale, AZ, USA 85258
Phone: 1-602-998-9331

The Upledger Institute, Inc. (CranioSacral Therapy™)
11211 Prosperity Farms Rd.
Palm Beach Gardens, FL, USA 33410
Phone: 1-800-233-5880

American Oriental Bodywork Therapy Association (AOBTA)
6801 Jericho Turnpike
Syosset, NY, USA 11791
Phone 1-516-364-5533

Healing Touch International, Inc.
12477 W. Cedar Drive, Suite #202
Lakewood, CO, USA 80228
Phone: 1-303-989-7982
Fax: 1-303-980-8683
http://www.healingtouch.net

Touch Research Institute
Dr. Tiffany Fields
Department of Pediatrics
University of Miami School of Medicine
P.O. Box 016820 (Dept. 820)
1601 NW 12th Avenue
Miami, FL, USA 33101
Phone: 1-305-243-6781
Fax: 1-305-243-6488
http://www.miami.edu/touch-research/

International Association of Infant Massage
Carla Steptoe, RNC, NNP, HN, CIMI
101 Hickory Drive
Ocean Springs, MS, USA 39564
Phone: 1-228-818-2704 Fax: 1-228-872-8044
e-mail for general information: cars@datasync.com
http://www.infantmassage.com

Nurse Healers—Professional Associates International
1211 Locust St.
Philadelphia, PA, USA 19107
Phone: 1-215-545-8079
nhpa@nursecominc.com
http://www.therapeutic-touch.org

American Holistic Nurses Association (AHNA)
P.O. Box 2130
Flagstaff, AZ, USA 86003-2130
Phone: 1-800-278-AHNA
e-mail: AHNA-Flag@flaglink.com
http://ahna.org

Resources for Further Learning:
Environment and Caring

Anthroposophical Nurses Association America
Gisela Franceschelli
Secretary, ANAA
Ghent, NY 12075
http://www.slip.net/~anaa

American Music Therapy Association, Inc.
8455 Colesville Road, Suite 1000
Silver Spring, MD, USA 20910
Phone: 1-301-589-3300
Fax: 1-301-589-5175
e-mail: info@musictherapy.org
www.musictherapy.org
www.musictherapy.ca

Horticultural Therapy
For international listing: http://www.hort.vt.edu//human/profht.html

Books listed by Elizabeth C. Miller Horticultural library in the USA
http://weber.u.washington.edu/~hortlib/booklists/hort.therapy.html

American Association of Naturopathic Physicians
601 Valley Street, Suite 105
Seattle, WA, USA 98109
Phone: 1-206-298-0126
Fax: 1-206-298-0129
www.healthy.net/clinic/therapy/naturopathic/
    Resource/index.htmlwww.naturopathics.com

General Council and Register of Naturopaths
GCRN, Goswell House
2 Goswell Road, Street
Somerset, BA16 0JG, UK
Phone: (01458) 840072
Fax: (01458) 840075
http://www.compulink.co.uk/~naturopathy/

American Alliance of Aromatherapy (AAOA)
PO Box 309
Depoe Bay, OR, USA 97341
Phone: 1-800-809-9850
aaoa@wcn.net

Mindy Green, MS—Aromatherapy
4133 Amber Street
Boulder, CO, USA 80304
Phone: 1-303-447-9552
(No correspondence courses)

R. Jane Buckle Associates LLC—Aromatherapy
P.O. Box 868
Hunter, NY, USA 12442
1–518-263-4402
rjbuckle@aol.com

National Association of Holistic Aromatherapy (NAHA)
Administrative Office
836 Hanely Industrial Court
St. Louis, MO, USA 63144
Phone: 1-888-ASK-NAHA
info@naha.org

For information about the American Alliance of Aromatherapy, the Alliance News Quarterly, *or the* International Journal of Aromatherapy, *call*
1-800-809-9850
Fax 1-800-809-9808
or write
American Alliance of Aromatherapy
P.O. Box 309
Depoe Bay, OR, USA 97341.

The Herb Society of America
9019 Kirtland Chardon Rd
Kirtland, OH, USA 44094
Phone: 1-440-256-0514
Fax: 1-440-256-0541
e-mail: herbs@herbsociety.org
http://www.herbsociety.org

The Friends of the Medicinal Herb Garden
c/o Botany Department
University of Washington
Box 355325
Seattle, WA, USA 98195–5325
Phone: 1-206-543-1126

American Botanical Council
P.O. Box 144345
Austin, TX, USA 78714-4345
Phone: 1-512-926-4900
Fax: 1-512-926-2345
www.herbalgram.org

Herb Research Foundation
1007 Pearl Street, Suite 200
Boulder, CO, USA 80302
Phone: 1-303-449-2265 (Office)
VoiceMail: 1-800-748-2617
Fax: 1-303-449-7849
www.herbs.org

The Richard and Hinda Rosenthal Center for Complementary & Alternative Medicine
Columbia University, College of Physicians & Surgeons
630 W. 168th Street, Box 75
New York, NY, USA 10032

American Herbalists Guild
P.O. Box 70
Roosevelt, UT, USA 84066
Phone: 1-435-722-8434
Fax: 1-435-722-8452
e-mail: ahgoffice@earthlink.net
http://www.healthy.net/herbalists/

Rocky Mountain Herbal Institute (RMHI)
Roger W. Wicke, PhD, Director of TCM herbal medicine education
c/o P.O. Box 579
Hot Springs, MT, USA 59845
Phone: 1-406-741-3811
http://www.rmhiherbal.org/

For international herbal medicine associations
http://www.herbnet.com/associations_p1.htm

Planetree Inc.
130 Division Street
Derby, CT, USA 06418
Phone: 1-203-732-1365
www.planetree.org

Resources for Further Learning: Nutrition

http://www.nutritionsciencenews.com

Center for Science in the Public Interest USA and Canada
http://www.cspinet.org/nah/

National Institutes of Health USA
Office of Dietary Supplements
http://www.odp.od.nih.gov/ods

American Association of Oriental Medicine
Phone: 1-610-266-1433
http://www.aaom.org

National Acupuncture and Oriental Medicine Alliance
Phone: 1-206-524-3511
76143.2061@compuserve.com

Diabetes
http://www.diabetes.rg
You can also call the American Diabetes Association at:
1-800-DIABETES (1-800-342-2383)

Or write:
American Diabetes Association
Attn: Customer Service
1660 Duke Street
Alexandria, VA, USA 22314

United States Department of Agriculture (USDA)
http://www.nal.usda.gov/fnic

Courses on food preparation and service can be found at most colleges and universities, often under home economics.

Council for Responsible Nutrition
1875 Eye Street, NW
Suite 400
Washington, DC, USA 20006-5409
Phone: 1-202-872-1488
Fax: 1-202-872-9594

American Academy of Nutrition
(accredited distance learning programs)
3408 Sausalito
Corona Del Mar, CA, USA 92625-1638
Fax: 1-949-760-1788
e-mail: aancal@aol.com
Also:
1212 Kenesaw
Knoxville, TN, USA 37919-7736
Fax: 1-423-524-8339
e-mail: aantn@aol.com
Phone: 1-800-290-4226
http://www.nutritioneducation.com/

Resources for Further Learning: Communication

Mindfulness Based Stress Reduction
http://www.mbsr.com/MBSR%20listings/director.htm
Lists International Education
http://www.ummed.edu/dept/Prevent.behav.med/faculty.html:
Faculty includes Jon-Kabat Zinn
Stress Reduction Clinic
University of Massachusetts Medical Center
55 Lake Avenue, North
Worcester, MA, USA 01655

*Further learning about communication techniques used in
Psychiatric/Mental Health nursing:*

American Psychiatric Nurses Association
1200 19th Street, NW
Suite 300
Washington, DC, USA 20036-2422
Phone: 1-202-857-1133
Fax: 1-202-223-4579
http://www.apna.org

Association of Child and Adolescent Psychiatric Nurses (ACAPN)
1211 Locust St.
Philadelphia, PA, USA 19107
Phone: 1-800-826-2950 or 1-215-545-2843
Fax: 1-215-545-8107
http://www.acapn.org

Dale Carnegie Training Institute
www.dale-carnegie.com

Toastmasters International
Phone: 1-800-993-7732 (for North America)
1-949-858-8255 (International)
www.toastmasters.org

Creative HealthCare Resources
1701 East 79th Street, Suite 1
Minneapolis, MN, USA 55425-1151
Phone: 1-800-264-3246
www.chcm.com

Institute of Heartmath
P.O. Box 1463
14700 West Park Ave.
Boulder Creek, CA, USA 95006
Phone: 1-831-338-8700
www.heartmath.com or www.heartmath.org

Search for books, videos, web sites, and college courses under the following categories: communication, customer service, and public speaking.

Resources for Further Learning:
Use of Energy in Nursing Practice

Society for Light Treatment and Biological Rhythms
Stephanie Argraves, Executive Director
842 Howard Avenue
New Haven, CT, USA 06519
Fax: 1-203-764-4324
e-mail: sltbr@yale.edu
http://www.websciences.org/sltbr/

Institute of Heartmath
14700 West Park Avenue
Boulder Creek, CA, USA 95006
Phone: 1-831-338-8500
Fax: 1-831-338-8500
e-mail: info@heartmath.org
http://www.heartmath.org/

Institute of Noetic Sciences
475 Gate Five Rd., Ste. 300
Sausalito, CA, USA 94965
Phone: 1-415-331-5650

Mind/Body Behavioral Medicine Clinic
Deaconess Hospital
Harvard Medical School
1 Deaconess Rd.
Boston, MA, USA 02215
Phone: 1-617-632-9530

Center for Mind-Body Medicine
5225 Connecticut Avenue, NW
Suite 414
Washington, DC, USA 20015
Phone: 1-202-966-7338
Fax: 1-202-966-2589
cmbm@mindspring.com

Institute for Frontier Science
Beverly Rubik, PhD
6114 LaSalle Avenue
Box 605
Oakland, CA, USA 94611
Phone: 1-510-531-5767
brubik@compuserve.com

Japanese research on biomagnetics
http://www.biomagnetic.com/journals/
    nakagawa.htm

B.K.S. Iyengar Yoga National Association of the United States
http://www.iyoga.com/IYNAUS/
Iyengar Yoga: certified teachers
http://www.iyoga.com/IYNAUS/certified
    teachers.html
United Kingdom: http://www.iyi.org.uk/

Integral Yoga International
R.R. 1
Box 1720
Buckingham, VA, USA 23902
Phone: 1-800-858-9642 (voice)
e-mail: Satchidananda Ashram home page
http://www.yogaville.org

International Tai Chi Federation
President G. Master Pablo Barboza
San Luis 3369 (CP 7600) Mar del Plata
Pcia de Buenos Aires, Argentina
Phone: (54-23)92-3303
Fax: (54-23) 75-655
e-mail: matcomp@statics.com.ar
http://www.sportscenter.com.ar/ITCF.html
Has listings of tai chi associations for many countries.

American Dance Therapy Association (ADTA) National Office
Business Hours: 8:30 A.M.–4:00 P.M. EST
Phone: 1-410-997-4040
Fax: 1-410-997-4048
e-mail: info@adta.org
http://www.adta.org

Academy for Guided Imagery, Inc.
P.O. Box 2070
Mill Valley, CA, USA 94942
Phone: 1-800-726-2070

For therapeutic touch information, please see resources in Chapter 7.

Index